Praise for *Navigating Your Healthcare Journey*

"The personal stories and lessons learned in *Navigating Your Healthcare Journey* highlight the importance of taking ownership of your health and of being your own advocate. It shares personal experiences of what can go wrong in this complicated, fragmented health care ecosystem when information isn't readily available to get the right care at the right time in the right place. *Navigating Your Healthcare Journey* is a wake-up call for patients and caregivers to proactively seek out resources to help understand treatment options and where to go for care."

BRIAN MARCOTTE   PAST CEO AND PRESIDENT, BUSINESS GROUP ON HEALTH; FORMER HONEYWELL EXECUTIVE

"Everyone needs a navigator for our $4 trillion, impossibly complicated healthcare system. Sadly, most patients never get the personal attention they so deserve. Enter Edwards and Rothkopf with the best navigation system I have ever seen. Everyone will be a patient, and everyone needs to read this book."

DAVID NASH, MD, MBA   FOUNDING DEAN EMERITUS, JEFFERSON UNIVERSITY COLLEGE OF POPULATION HEALTH; DR. RAYMOND C. AND DORIS N GRANDON PROFESSOR; EDITOR-IN-CHIEF, *AMERICAN JOURNAL OF MEDICAL QUALITY AND POPULATION HEALTH*

"The book is excellent, and I say that with the highest praise. It is easy to read, clear, and understandable. I liked the format—filled with enough information and great stories which are engaging and thought-provoking. I can't tell you which chapter I liked the best because they are all great."

CAROL ORAVEC, RN

"*Navigating Your Healthcare Journey* is the go-to practical guide for patients and their families traversing the often tortuous terrain known as the U.S. healthcare experience."

SARIA (CARTER) SACCOCIO, MD, MHA, FAAFP
CHIEF MEDICAL OFFICER, CAREMORE HEALTH, EAST REGION

"*Navigating Your Healthcare Journey* is filled with useful and understandable information about how our healthcare system works. This practical guide should be required reading for healthcare management students and medical, nursing, and other health professional students. It is refreshing to see things from the view of the patient and understand in human terms the challenges they face with our healthcare system each and every day!"

AMANDA HOPKINS TIRRELL, MBA, FACHE
PRESIDENT AND FOUNDER, HOPKINS TIRRELL & ASSOCIATES, LLC

"*Navigating Your Healthcare Journey* is a compilation of the expertise, compassion, care, and the lived experience of these passionate authors. Their years in the service of others at all levels of our healthcare system delivers a skillful meshing of science, storytelling, education and empowerment.

"Both comprehensive and concise, this well researched guide is the ideal companion as one journeys, as patient and advocate, through the morass that is healthcare in this country today. It provides the tools to be in action in addressing healthcare decisions with awareness, focus and confidence. You will refer to this guide often as a trusted resource—its format is readable, informative and actionable."

MAGDA BARINI-GARCIA, MD, MPH   HEALTH POLICY PHYSICIAN; FORMER SENIOR MEDICAL ADVISOR ON MINORITY HEALTH AND HEALTH DISPARITIES AND QUALITY, HEALTH RESOURCES AND SERVICES ADMINISTRATION (HRSA) CENTER FOR QUALITY; CAPTAIN, UNITED STATES PUBLIC HEALTH SERVICE (RETIRED)

"*Navigating Your Healthcare Journey* is essential reading for anyone trying to access, coordinate, or live with a chronic condition. I wish our healthcare system did not need such a book. Yet, it desperately does. Our healthcare system is confusing, chaotic, and clunky, rather than coordinated and compassionate. Ms. Rothkopf and Dr. Edwards bring tremendous lived experience, profound passion, and compassion to help ensure those needing care can be as healthy as they can be. Their recommendations are grounded in science, ruthlessly practical, and provide deep insights for all."

PETER PRONOVOST, MD, PHD CHIEF CLINICAL TRANSFORMATION OFFICER, UNIVERSITY HOSPITALS; FORMER SVP, PATIENT SAFETY AND QUALITY, JOHNS HOPKINS; FOUNDER AND FORMER DIRECTOR, JOHNS HOPKINS ARMSTRONG INSTITUTE FOR PATIENT SAFETY & QUALITY

"This highly readable, engaging book provides a useful compass to anyone trying to navigate the complexities of our healthcare system."

DAVID B. HELLMANN, MD, MACP ALIKI PERROTI PROFESSOR OF MEDICINE, JOHNS HOPKINS UNIVERSITY SCHOOL OF MEDICINE; DIRECTOR, JOHNS HOPKINS CENTER FOR INNOVATIVE MEDICINE

Navigating Your
Healthcare Journey

Navigating Your Healthcare Journey

**LESSONS LEARNED
TO GET THE CARE
YOU NEED & DESERVE**

Charlene Rothkopf, MA · Z. Colette Edwards, MD, MBA

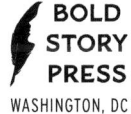

BOLD
STORY
PRESS

WASHINGTON, DC

Bold Story Press, Washington, DC 20016
www.boldstorypress.com

Copyright © 2023 by Charlene Rothkopf, MA and Z. Colette Edwards, MD MBA

All rights reserved. No part of this book may be reproduced or used in any manner without written permission of the copyright owner except for the use of quotations in a book review. Requests for permission or further information should be submitted through info@boldstorypress.com.

The stories in this book are true. In some cases, the patients requested their real names be used. Others wanted to maintain anonymity, and therefore their names were changed.

This book is written and published with a goal of providing accurate information relevant to the topics. However, ensuring all information provided is entirely accurate and up to date at all times is not possible. Therefore, the authors and publisher accept no responsibility for inaccuracies, errors, misstatements, inconsistencies, or omissions and specifically disclaim any liability, loss, or risk, personal, professional, or otherwise, which may be incurred as a consequence, directly or indirectly, of the use and/or application of any of the contents of this book.

It is published and sold with the understanding that the authors and publisher are not engaged in rendering legal, medical, or other professional services by reason of their authorship or publication of this work. The authors and the book do not provide medical advice, diagnosis, or treatment, nor recommend or endorse any specific tests, medical professionals, products, procedures, opinions, or other information that may be mentioned. Reliance on any information provided is solely at your own risk.

Always seek the advice of your physician or other qualified healthcare provider with any questions you may have regarding a medical condition. Never disregard professional medical advice or delay in seeking it because of something you have read in this book. If you think you may have a medical emergency, call your doctor or 911 immediately. If medical, legal, or other expert assistance is required, the services of a competent professional person should be sought.

Any views expressed are of those of the authors and do not represent the views of their employers, past or present.

First edition: May 2023

Library of Congress Control Number: 2023905092
ISBN: 978-1-954805-48-4 (paperback)
ISBN: 978-1-954805-49-1 (ebook)

Author photo for Charlene Rothkopf by Tamzin B. Smith Portrait Photography
Author photo for Z. Colette Edwards by Evan Cohen Photography

Printed in the United States of America
10 9 8 7 6 5 4 3 2 1

Our book is dedicated to:

My husband, David, and my children, Michael and Emily, who supported me throughout my healthcare journey and, along with their families, continue to bring joy to my life.

My dear friends and relatives for their enduring gifts of kindness and compassion.

The many devoted healthcare professionals—doctors, nurses, and administrators—who provided invaluable care and expertise along the way and continue to do so.

Charlene

My parents, E. Zeno Edwards, MD and Mattie S. Edwards, EdD, for their unconditional love and unerring support. They were very much ahead of their time, and their pioneering spirit, integrity, and empathetic and inclusive worldview have made all the difference in my life.

My sister, Tanise I. Edwards, MD, who has been the very best friend and confidante one could hope to have. Knowing I have her as my travel companion through both the ups and downs life brings to us all is a source of comfort (and fun!) and wonderful shared memories in the making. And writing a chapter for her book years ago opened the door and brought inspiration to writing books myself.

The many patients I have had the unique honor and pleasure to serve. Their strength, grace, and trust have enriched my life immeasurably and provided a sense of purpose, satisfaction, and contentment that is difficult to put into words.

Colette

Contents

	Preface	xiii
INTRODUCTION	Our Stories	1
	Charlene's Story	1
	Colette's Story	23
CHAPTER 1	Taking Charge of Your Health	33
CHAPTER 2	Embracing a Healthier Lifestyle	51
CHAPTER 3	Choosing the Type of Doctor You Need	81
CHAPTER 4	Partnering with Your Doctor	103
CHAPTER 5	Coordinating Care	125
CHAPTER 6	Having a Baby	141
CHAPTER 7	Deciding Where to Go When a Medical Need Arises	163
CHAPTER 8	Maintaining Your Emotional Health	177
CHAPTER 9	Dealing with Mental Illness	193
CHAPTER 10	Facing Health Disparities	211
CHAPTER 11	Paying for Healthcare	237
CHAPTER 12	Preparing for the End of Life	275
	Epilogue	301
	Acknowledgments	311
	Resources	315
	Guide to Acronyms & Abbreviations	327
	Endnotes	333
	About the Authors	345

Preface

I learned a long time ago the wisest thing I can do is be on my own side, be an advocate for myself and others like me.

MAYA ANGELOU

Navigating the healthcare system in the United States can be one of the most difficult and complicated journeys you can take. It can be confusing and daunting for the savviest individual, even for those with a medical background. When people are faced with a chronic health problem, an acute event, or the prospect of a life-threatening condition, it is natural to feel scared, vulnerable, and overwhelmed. Given the complexity and fragmentation of the medical environment, it can be challenging to find the right resources and support.

While the U.S. has many of the best healthcare professionals, facilities, and researchers in the world, the cost of accessing those resources can be beyond reach for many.

And the recent COVID-19 pandemic has highlighted the many long-standing inequities that exist across the country, particularly among people of color, those in the LGBTQIA+ (lesbian, gay, bisexual, transgender, queer, intersex, asexual, and others) community, those living with a disability, and those with a lower socioeconomic status in both urban and rural areas.

You may be wondering how this book came to be.

Both of us completed the graduate certificate program in health and wellness coaching at the Maryland University of Integrative Health. We first met as participants on a panel to discuss the coaching program with prospective students and just hit it off. We then continued to work together, offering a series of breakfast seminars to executive women, including "Leading with Authenticity" and "The Art & Science of Healthy Aging."

Both of us had dealt with the healthcare system professionally. Charlene has worked as a director of health and welfare benefits and vice president for a global hospitality company, as a senior human resource executive for a national real estate company, and currently as an executive coach and management consultant. She also volunteered as co-chair of a patient and family advisory council for a major academic medical system. Colette has worked as a practicing physician, healthcare consultant, coach, and health plan medical director, and as a corporate medical executive for employee health and well-being at a Fortune 50 company.

We have also dealt with the healthcare system personally—one as a patient (Charlene) and the other as a practicing physician and caregiver to parents (Colette). These experiences took us deep into the reality of the many complexities that all too often are encountered by patients. In this book, we will share our own personal experiences, along with those of others who were eager to convey their perspectives and granted us permission to tell their stories. The patients and caregivers we interviewed represent the real-life experiences of a diverse group of individuals—age, race/ethnicity, geographic locale, socioeconomic status, education level, and access to healthcare resources. While some may have had more education, financial advantage, or support networks, all struggled with navigating the U.S. healthcare system in some way.

Each chapter begins with a story, which is followed by "Lessons Learned," based on the patient's and/or caregiver's experiences. Next is "What You Need to Know," including an overview of the topic, pertinent data, and some helpful checklists. At the end of each chapter, we offer suggestions for actions you can take under the heading "So, What Can You Do Now?"

Our goal is to help you be more confident and develop the self-advocacy skills needed to navigate the healthcare system and obtain the care you need and deserve. While many of the chapter topics are interrelated, each one covers a specific healthcare issue and can be read in the sequence that is most relevant to you.

In this book, we offer no medical advice, nor do we advocate for one type of treatment, clinician, or institution over another. We greatly respect the many selfless and dedicated healthcare professionals, as well as the incredible technical advances and resources that are available in the U.S. The pandemic has shone a light on the healthcare heroes in our midst, and we honor those who have been on the front lines in the battle against COVID-19.

We also recognize that medicine will continue to be both an art and a science. It takes a true partnership between healthcare professionals and the patients/caregivers to produce optimal outcomes. It takes a willingness, on the part of both the clinicians and the patients/caregivers, to ask questions, listen, and work together with respect and compassion.

Put simply, our hope is to help you, the patient or caregiver, become empowered with greater knowledge and the confidence to act as a strong advocate for yourself and your loved ones throughout your unique healthcare journey.

INTRODUCTION

Our Stories

To know even one life has breathed easier because you have lived. This is to have succeeded.

RALPH WALDO EMERSON

We have chosen to begin the book with our stories, as they were the primary impetus and motivation for our writing. Our experiences—as a patient with an extended and complicated illness and as a physician who has tried to approach patients with empathy and compassion—formed the basis for much of the book's content. Here are our stories.

CHARLENE'S STORY

January 2008

I was a busy human resources executive of a national public company. At the beginning of every year, I would schedule an off-site team meeting to determine our goals and priorities for the year. Following a successful planning meeting, we all went to dinner and exchanged post-holiday "Secret Santa" gifts. It was a fantastic day.

I arrived home at about 8:45 p.m. and greeted my husband, who was watching TV. I changed my clothes and began to check my emails for the day. While at the computer, my left hand suddenly began to cramp. I called to my husband, "Something is wrong with my hand!"

"Oh, it's probably just a cramp," he responded nonchalantly. "Let me stretch it out." He tried to pry open my fingers, but my left hand wouldn't open. Immediately the spasm worked its way up my left arm, and, in seconds, my entire left side tightened. I could sense the blood draining from the left side of my face. As my knees began to buckle, my last thought was, *I think I'm having a stroke. Call 911*, but the words never came. I blacked out and collapsed into my husband's arms.

While holding me in one hand, my husband dialed 911 with the other. His cell phone had almost no battery power left, and he was frantically hoping that it would last through the call. Then he laid me gently on the floor and waited for the ambulance.

I remember waking to the EMTs (emergency medical technicians) in my house. Sitting me on a chair, one EMT began to ask questions. "What's your name?" "Where are you?" "What's today's date?" He asked me to smile and noticed that the left side of my mouth was not turning up like the other side. I was alert and lucid, but my hands were shaking. They strapped me onto a gurney and wheeled me out the front door into the ambulance. They radioed the emergency room that I was on the way, while my husband followed in his car.

I was quickly whisked to the MRI (magnetic resonance imaging) machine for the first of several MRIs that would follow. The claustrophobic chamber, the loud clanging noise, and the inability to move were anxiety-provoking, but I kept my eyes shut and breathed slowly.

At some point after midnight, the ER doctor entered my room with the results. "Well, the good news is that you didn't have a stroke," he stated rather matter-of-factly. "The bad news is that you have a brain tumor. You had a focal seizure that was caused by the tumor."

"It's called a meningioma," he said. "Because of where it's located, you're going to need surgery to remove it."

"A what?" I asked. "Surgery? How soon? In the next few months?"

"No, you can't wait that long," he replied. "You'll have to have surgery as soon as possible. You can talk with the neurosurgeon when he gets here. You'll be admitted to the hospital for the night."

"Call my office in the morning," I told my husband. "Tell them I won't be coming in."

I knew my staff was highly capable, and I was confident the work would carry on as usual. Amazing how suddenly one's priorities change!

There wasn't a room available at the hospital that evening, so I stayed in the emergency room. I wasn't about to sleep anyway; there were so many thoughts racing through my head. *What about the kids? I have to let them know what happened. Will I live through this? Is it cancer? Will I live to see my children get married, and will I ever spend time with my grandchildren?*

At 4:00 a.m., a bed became available. As they wheeled me off the elevator, I noticed I was being taken to the oncology wing. *Oh no, I thought, maybe I do have brain cancer.*

The nurse arrived to ask for my name and medical history and to take my temperature and blood pressure. "Do you have a living will?" the nurse said to me. "I have to ask you that."

"I do, but I haven't looked at it in a long time." The possibility that I might not survive hit me hard.

The nurse was efficient and very kind. She had worked the night shift at the hospital for over thirty years. This was the first of many encounters with a special group of people who are incredibly dedicated and committed to taking care of others. I began to appreciate the compassionate nature of the nursing staff and what they do day after day.

At 6:30 a.m., the neurosurgeon on call came to my room. He repeated that I had a meningioma, which is more common in women than men. While there's no certainty, most of these tumors are benign. But I needed to have it removed as soon as possible. "These types of tumors are slow growing," he explained. "It must have been there for a long time—and they are often asymptomatic."

"What causes it?" I asked.

"We don't know," he responded. "There are many theories, but none have been proven."

"Where exactly is the tumor?" I asked.

"It's about here," he said, pointing to the top of my head, slightly right of center, about parallel to my right ear. "The good news is that it's at the top, not deep inside the brain. If you had to have a brain tumor, this is the one to have, since it's most easily operable and usually benign." I felt somewhat relieved but still anxious.

"Will you have to shave my whole head?" I asked sheepishly.

"No," he said, "We usually don't have to. Just a strip of hair will be removed where the incision is made."

He prescribed Keppra, an anti-seizure medication, and a steroid for the swelling. I had to schedule surgery quickly.

Finding a surgeon

During the next week, I went into high-task mode. I contacted anyone who had been through a similar experience and requested information about the best neurosurgeons and hospitals. Although I never thought of myself as a great networker, friends and family members proved to be invaluable resources.

A friend who worked in the radiology department of the hospital knew a team of neurosurgeons and recommended one who was well regarded by the hospital staff. Through this friend, we obtained a computer disk copy and a set of hard copies of the MRI results to bring to my doctor visits.

Then we learned of someone recently diagnosed with brain cancer who was being treated by the head of the neurosurgery department at a well-known hospital about an hour away. We were able to obtain the doctor's name, phone number, and email address to send him the MRI results.

Another friend suggested I speak to a woman who had been treated by the local neurosurgeon. She told me that even though the surgery had been successful, she had suffered through some post-operative blood clots and had fallen while she was in the hospital. I realized that, while selecting the right surgeon was very important, the post-operative care was critical as well. If the hospital was not sufficiently staffed or equipped to attend to a patient's needs after the surgery, additional problems could occur.

But the best connection came from another friend who had a contact at a cancer foundation in the area. Although we never met face-to-face, the contact was able to arrange an appointment with the highly recommended chief neurosurgeon at a prominent hospital. "He has helped so many people that I know," she said.

The following week, I met with the local neurosurgeon first. The doctor was excellent and spent over an hour with my husband and me explaining what was going to happen and answering our questions. I cried through most of the consultation. There was no viable option other than surgery, as the tumor had already grown too large.

He explained the risks of the surgery. The tumor was very close to the sagittal sinus, a critical vein in the brain; if touched during surgery, the result could be fatal. The tumor was also positioned close to the motor strip, which controls the mobility of one's arms and legs. The pressure and inflammation of the tumor on the right side of my brain had caused the seizure on the left side of my body.

We talked about the timing of the surgery and his availability. He was booked and would have to make room on his schedule to fit me in.

"What about the hospital and the post-operative care?" I asked.

"Well, the hospital is very good, but there is a nursing shortage everywhere," he responded.

I appreciated his honesty but was somewhat concerned. I didn't want to be in the hospital bed after surgery and not have a nurse available to respond to my call button. Although I'm sure he was an excellent surgeon, I was concerned about the staffing shortage at the hospital. On the other hand, the hospital was about fifteen minutes from our home and very convenient. My husband and I drove home discussing this local option.

Two days later, we drove an hour to the other large hospital. Upon entering the main door, I was overwhelmed by the enormity of the facility. It was a city within a city. Groups of people were moving in all directions—young interns busily chatting with each other, visitors with name tags trying to keep pace with their guides, and patients from foreign countries attempting to find their way through the maze.

As the paper security band was fastened around my wrist, my eyes welled with tears. I turned to my husband and cried, "I don't think I can do this. It's too much."

Maria, the woman at the registration desk, sensed my anxiety and greeted me with a big smile. I gave her my name, and she responded, "Yes, you're already in our system, and we're expecting you. I even know your birthday. It's April twentieth, isn't it?"

"Yes," I replied sheepishly, not wanting her to see my watery eyes and blotchy face.

She handed me a plastic card that would be my ID for use in every department of the hospital so that all the billing could be centrally coordinated. She directed us to the neurosurgery department for my appointment and wished us good luck. I thanked her and returned the smile, wiping my eyes with a tissue.

Arriving at the neurosurgery area, we were asked to sign in and take a number.

My number was called, and we were escorted to a small examining room. The first person to enter was a senior resident. He reviewed the MRI results with us, confirming what the other neurosurgeon had told us, and explained the procedure, the risks, and what to expect.

The next person to speak to us was a neurological nurse who was doing research as part of her training. She said she would be following my case before, during, and after the surgery. As this was a teaching hospital, I was impressed not only by the intellectual caliber of the individuals who spoke with us but also by their commitment to learning as much as they could about me and my situation.

When the neurosurgeon finally came in, I was immediately struck by his compassion and optimism. Like the other neurosurgeon, he reiterated that surgery was my only option, but he reassured me I would get through this with flying colors. While he reviewed all the risks, he comforted me by stating the one or two millimeters between the tumor and the sagittal sinus was "like a mile" to him.

After listening to his assessment of my case and the procedure that I would go through, I had a few critical questions. With as much frankness as I could muster, I said, "I know I'm not the most complicated or challenging case you will see, and that you have patients with a lot more serious tumors, but it's still brain surgery. Will you be the one conducting the surgery, or are you going to hand me off to one of your associates?"

"I'll be doing the surgery, but I will also have two other neurosurgeons assisting me," he replied. "They are both in their final year of residency with us and will be practicing at Harvard and other fine institutions when they leave in June. They have years of experience in this field and are two of the most brilliant physicians I've ever worked with. The anesthesiologist is excellent, and the nursing team is specifically trained in this area."

I felt reassured by his answer and then asked, "This hospital is such a huge place; how can you ensure that I won't get lost in the bureaucratic maze?"

The neurosurgeon broke into a grin and responded, "The surgery may take anywhere from three to nine hours, and you will be my only patient that day. I will see you the day before your surgery, in the ICU [intensive care unit] after it's over, and when you come back to see me ten days later. In the interim, I will be phoning in to check on your progress during your recovery."

"What about the nursing shortage?" I inquired, remembering what the other doctor had said.

"What nursing shortage?" he replied. "We have a long line of nurses waiting to work for us. We have a twenty-two-room neurosurgical ICU with nurses specifically trained to handle post-operative brain surgery and two floors of step-down neurosurgical care with staff skilled in this specialty as well."

With that information, I decided to move forward as quickly as possible. We scheduled the surgery for the following Wednesday morning, with pre-op on Tuesday.

Talking to the family

Although I maintained a positive and hopeful outlook, there was always a chance I might not make it out of surgery alive. Would I get to see my family again? How do you say goodbye to your children? How do I tell them everything in my heart in such a short amount of time? I decided it was time to do just that.

Our son and daughter, both in their twenties and out of college, were living on their own, leading independent lives. After a few failed attempts, they were able to come to the house at the same time. I turned off the TV and asked them to put away their cell phones. "I need to talk to you both," I said, realizing this was far more difficult for them to hear than it was for me to say.

"I want you both to know I love you more than anything in the world," I began. "If anything happens to me, I want you to know that. And when I come out of surgery, you and Dad are the ones I want to see. No matter who is at the hospital, I want to see your faces first."

"If something happens to me," I proceeded, "you need to know where the will is and what I want to happen. First, Dad and I are going to update our wills, and everything is to be split fifty-fifty. You are adults now, so we're not going to specify who gets what. You're just going to have to talk with each other and work things out. No fighting over stuff." I showed them where the wills were stored, along with the name of the estate attorney with whom we worked.

"And I want to apologize for any time when I didn't hug you enough or kiss you enough while you were growing up. You know I always loved you both, but sometimes I didn't always express it. Please remember that." The kids didn't say much, but I knew they were listening.

Something was different after that talk—nothing big, just subtle changes. The invisible wall between us had begun to crumble. It wasn't until after the surgery that I could really see the maturity in my children I had never seen before. They began to talk more with me and with each other and took care of me in so many ways after the surgery. The silver lining in this whole ordeal is that it probably helped our family grow closer.

Gathering the necessary documents

Since we hadn't updated our will in about ten years, I called the estate attorney and set up an appointment to see him, two days before the surgery. During our meeting, the attorney gave me three documents to take to the hospital. Due to the HIPAA (Health Insurance Portability and Accountability

Act) privacy of information legislation, the first document allowed for the release of my medical information to my husband and children. The other documents included an updated living will and a healthcare power of attorney that gave my husband and children the decision-making power to withdraw life support interventions that would keep me alive if there was no possibility of recovery.

The surgery and early recovery

We arrived at the hospital at 5:30 a.m. Neither of us had slept much the night before, knowing we had to leave the house by 4:30 a.m. When we entered the main registration area, Maria was again there to greet us. It felt reassuring to see a familiar face.

"Don't you ever go home?" I asked her.

"No, I pretty much live here," she replied with a smile, and gave us directions to the surgery prep area.

Once upstairs, I was escorted into the pre-op area. I put on a hospital gown, and IV (intravenous) tubes were inserted into my arms. My stoic facade began to crumble. My husband came in and took the bag of my clothes. We talked briefly with the anesthesiologist about what was going to happen next. Then I was wheeled down the hall to the operating room. I don't remember anything else, as the anesthesia took effect almost immediately.

The surgery lasted about five hours. The entire tumor was removed, and fortunately it was benign. However, it had attached to many of the blood vessels, and I had lost a lot of blood in the process.

As the anesthesia was wearing off, my head was in a deep cloud, and all I wanted to do was sleep. My throat was raw from the anesthesia tube, and my mouth felt incredibly dry. The doctor had warned me to expect that. The doctors asked me my name and where I was.

"My throat hurts," I said, still in a fog, and then dropped back off to sleep. When I finally awoke, my daughter came in and began to spoon-feed me ice chips to soothe my throat. The ice chips were a welcomed relief.

As I regained more consciousness, I recognized the rest of the family who had come to the hospital. Although my head was wrapped in a gauze turban with drainage tubes coming out the back, I felt no pain. The biggest annoyance was the IV in my arm. I was on intravenous fluids and a heavy dose of steroids to keep the swelling down. With each dose of steroids, I would feel a burning sensation and couldn't wait to get rid of the IV in my bruised arm.

The neurosurgeon checked on me that afternoon. "The pain from the sore throat and IV is normal," he said, "and you came through the surgery with flying colors." I would have to stay in the ICU that night. The surgeon answered questions from the family, and we appreciated his kindness. Outside the room, the neurosurgeon thanked my husband for choosing the hospital to have the surgery, and my husband replied, "No pun intended, but it was a no-brainer."

That evening, all my visitors went home, and I spent the night trying to get comfortable.

The next shift was staffed by a young, male ICU nurse who was very attentive and efficient. He propped pillows under my knees or under my head and kept me stocked with ice chips for my throat.

At one point during the night, the catheter backed up, and I woke up in a pool of urine in my bed. I rang the call bell. With great efficiency, he proceeded to roll me from one side to the other, strip the bedsheets and replace them with new, dry ones. He used baby wipes to clean me and readjusted the catheter. From that point on, he very closely monitored the fluids coming out of the catheter.

When my family arrived the next day, I was so glad to see them. At one point, I was beginning to get hungry, and a cousin was able to obtain a tray of food for me. It was so good to taste real food again, as I hadn't eaten since the day before the surgery. She even managed to find a stash of graham crackers and brought me some apple juice. My daughter returned to cut up the food on my meal tray and to feed it to me. She was remarkable! My son came every day to check on me as well. My husband was exhausted; I could see this was all taking a toll on him. How fortunate I was to have my family there!

By the second day in the ICU, I was eager to get up and move around.

The gifts of family and friends

I was overwhelmed and humbled by the huge outpouring of love and support by everyone who heard about my diagnosis and surgery. The news spread quickly, and many longtime friends called and emailed me, literally from around the world. Flowers, cards, and other goodies arrived daily. My office arranged to have several meals delivered to my home.

A truly special gift was from a friend who collected all the email addresses of our friends and family. Her emails updated everyone on my progress, and she became the conduit of information. The likelihood of another seizure is more pronounced during those first two weeks following surgery, so she organized a schedule of shifts for people to stay at my house during the first two weeks at home. That way, with my husband at work, I wouldn't have to be alone.

During my recovery, my family supported me in so many ways. My daughter took me to lunch and to run errands before returning to work. My son called me daily. My sister-in-law stocked my refrigerator full of food. My niece and nephew visited and drove me to my physical therapy sessions. A cousin's visit truly boosted my spirits!

Many friends and family members wanted to help, but sometimes they didn't know what to do. What I learned to appreciate was that each person had individual gifts to offer, and the gifts reflected his or her unique strengths. Whether it was a friend's master organizing skills, a colleague's empathy, a neighbor's prayers, a sister-in-law's cooking, or a cousin's no-time-for-self-pity approach, they all offered generous and humbling gifts. I cherished whatever people had to offer and accepted it all, with much gratitude. The incredible outpouring of support allowed me to realize how much my family and friends meant to me and how much their support aided my recovery. With this realization, I wrote a heartfelt letter to the neurosurgeon expressing my appreciation to him and to the wonderful nursing staff.

September 2008 to January 2009

I was able to resume work after a three-month hiatus, and life seemed to go back to normal. In the fall of 2008, however, I noticed a wound on my head that refused to heal and repeatedly scabbed over. Subsequent MRIs showed no evidence of any tumor growth, and the neurosurgeon suggested we watch it for a while. I continued to see the neurosurgeon on an outpatient basis, but, as the wound still did not heal by December, I was referred to a plastic surgeon at the hospital. He scheduled the follow-up surgery for January 2009, exactly one year following the original surgery.

The 2009 surgery was the complete opposite experience from the 2008 surgery. I arrived at the hospital at 5:30 a.m., as instructed, and waited for the pre-op procedures to begin. No one came to check on me or even to acknowledge that my surgery was about to occur.

While lying in bed, I heard my neurosurgeon's voice speaking to a patient in the next bed behind the curtain. He wasn't aware that I was in pre-op, as the plastic surgeon had not communicated with him about my surgery that morning.

Finally, after I made several inquiries, the plastic surgeon arrived, and I was wheeled into surgery. Although I had been one of the first to arrive in the pre-op area, I was one of the last to be taken into surgery.

I awoke in the recovery room unaware of what procedure had been performed. The recovery room experience was less than ideal. Once again, my throat was raw and sore from the anesthesia tube, and I begged for someone to give me ice chips to soothe my throat and wet my lips. My husband was allowed to visit me for only a few minutes at a time. During most of my recovery room stay, I was on my own.

Waiting for a patient room to become available was a long ordeal. After making repeated requests, I was finally taken to a semi-private room on a different floor than the year prior. This floor seemed terribly understaffed. While the nurses tried hard, they couldn't keep up with the requests from all the patients. If I rang the bell for assistance to go to the bathroom, it would take twenty to thirty minutes before someone arrived, if anyone ever did.

Eventually, the plastic surgeon arrived to explain what had happened during the surgery. In the initial 2008 surgery, he explained, the bone at the top of my head—which had been removed and later reinserted after the tumor was excised—had become infected. This was why the surgical site was not healing properly. During this second surgery, the plastic surgeon had removed the infected bone and implanted a titanium plate in its place. I would need to stay in the hospital that night and could likely go home the next day.

That evening, a young nurse on the night shift entered my room. She seemed new and inexperienced. She approached my bed with a chart in her hand and began to review my allergies to specific medications. "No," I responded. "I'm not allergic to those medicines."

"Oops," she replied. "That's your roommate's chart." After she left, my roommate and I looked at each other. We agreed that this was going to be a long night—and it was.

The next morning, the doctor said I could be discharged. While the decision was made by 10:00 a.m., it took all day to leave the hospital. We waited hours for prescriptions from the infectious disease doctors and for the discharge papers to be issued. Between the neurosurgeon, the plastic surgeon, and the two infectious disease doctors, I wasn't sure who was truly in charge of my care. Although all the physicians were very cordial and professional, it seemed to me they couldn't agree on what to prescribe or the appropriate course of action.

Finally, at about 7:00 p.m., after waiting over an hour for a wheelchair to be brought to my room, my husband and I decided to walk out of the hospital on our own. On the way out, we saw a long row of available wheelchairs stacked by the entrance to the hospital. So, with the drainage tube still attached to the back of my head, we walked out of the hospital to our car. I needed to go home and rest. Two days later, I returned to have the drainage tube removed.

February 2009 to July 2009

The following six months became a nightmare. The incision on my head repeatedly opened to the point that tiny holes appeared at the top of my head and the titanium mesh insert was visible to the naked eye. Thirty days after the January 2009 surgery, I endured a follow-up visit to the plastic surgeon's office to stitch up the holes in my head even tighter this time. "It can't open now," he told me. But the surgical site continued to open. This time, however, I felt even more pain as the tight stitches were coming apart. With each footstep, I felt a sharp twinge of pain in my scalp.

I called the plastic surgeon again, and he scheduled a third surgery to repair the wound. But this third surgery proved futile as well, and the incision continued to open.

Repeated calls and emails to the plastic surgeon were fruitless. He sent me an email suggesting that I should "just relax in a warm bath, and don't worry if it's not oozing." I was totally frustrated.

By June 2009, a friend suggested I go to a wound care center at a nearby hospital. Upon examination, the doctor was appalled at the opening of my surgical incision and took photographs of the three holes at the top of my head. She said to me, "You shouldn't be walking around like this. You are at risk of infection." I requested that she call the neurosurgeon who performed the original surgery because I was having no luck in getting the matter addressed myself. She did so and forwarded the photographs to him.

Later that day, after returning to work, I received a phone call from the neurosurgeon's office requesting I come back to be admitted to the hospital that evening.

Medication

It is important to note that during this six-month period, I was being treated by two infectious disease doctors. Although they were cordial and professional, the experience was frustrating. To control the infection, I was given a series of antibiotics to fight a variety of bacteria, even though two of the bacteria naturally occur on one's skin and hair. Because I'm allergic to penicillin, they prescribed clindamycin. Other medications were suggested to combat the infection during this time; at one point, I said to the doctors, "Before I take this, why don't we check first to see if it is sensitive to the particular type of bacteria at the surgical site?"

"Good idea," said one of the infectious disease doctors.

I took these oral antibiotics for several months, and eventually my intestinal tract became upset. Since the surgical site was still not staying closed, they decided to prescribe home infusions of vancomycin intravenously through a PICC (peripherally inserted central catheter) line, a long, thin tube inserted through a vein in the arm.

After the PICC line was inserted at the nearby hospital, a home health nurse arrived at my door with two weeks' worth of vancomycin for me to self-administer. As the nurse administered the first dosage of vancomycin at my kitchen table, a rash broke out and my entire body turned red and itchy. I quickly was given an EpiPen injection to counteract the rash.

"Take out the PICC line," I insisted. "I won't be able to give myself these infusions while I'm alone at home and my husband is at work. What if this same reaction occurs again?" The nurse removed the PICC line, and I slept for about fifteen hours afterward.

With the ongoing prescriptions of antibiotics, the plastic surgeon made an offhand comment at one of the office visits that I was liable to get *C. diff.* I didn't know what that was at the time, nor did he offer to explain it to me. I later realized that *C. diff (Clostridium difficile)* is a gastrointestinal infection resulting from an overgrowth of bacteria after antibiotic treatment; it can be fatal if not treated.

In fact, I was on a visit to New York City with my family when the first bout of *C. diff* surfaced. Early on a Sunday morning before any of the stores opened, my husband and I were walking down Fifth Avenue. Suddenly and with great urgency, I had to go to the bathroom, but no place was open. I saw a man opening the employee entrance of a restaurant and raced to the door before it closed behind him. I asked for the restroom, ignoring his objection that the restaurant wasn't open yet. I found the restroom but did not make it to the toilet in time. I valiantly tried to clean up the floor and walked to the exit sheepishly. On the way out, the manager complained that I shouldn't have been in there. We made it back to the hotel to change and rest. When I returned home, my gastroenterologist gave me a prescription of Flagyl and saved me from any future recurrence.

Solving the mystery

After six months of antibiotics and two failed plastic surgeries, I was readmitted to the hospital. I arrived at 9:00 p.m. and was told not to eat anything since they might have to do surgery the next day. I waited throughout the next morning and afternoon without any food or fluids. I sat in the hospital room with my husband, not sure what was happening and with no word from any doctor. Finally, at 3:00 p.m., I called the neurosurgeon's office and asked, "Is anyone going to come by to see me today?"

At about 4:45 p.m., the neurosurgeon brought the chief of reconstructive surgery to my room to examine my head. Having seen this problem before, he immediately said, "You don't have an infection. Your head is rejecting the titanium plate. You're not going to like what I have to say, but it's the only solution. You will need surgery to remove the existing plate, wait six months for the bone to heal, and then undergo another surgery to insert a new titanium plate. During the six-month healing period, you will have to wear a protective helmet to avoid any injury to your brain, given there will be no bone and no plate to protect it."

Although I was devastated to learn that I had to endure two more surgeries, at least I had a clear diagnosis and a plan to move forward. "How could I be sure the second plate would work?" I asked. The reconstructive surgeon assured me he had seen this before and knew how to implant the titanium plate so that it would hold. I felt I was finally in good hands with the chief of reconstructive surgery in charge, and the next surgery was scheduled within thirty days.

I learned that the neurosurgeon had been unaware of all I had been through over the past six months. There had been little to no communication across departments, and no one had been coordinating my care during this time. My treatment across three departments—neurosurgery, plastic surgery, and infectious disease—had been fragmented and disjointed. It was evident the physicians had not communicated with each other in the handling of my case. I had incorrectly assumed that they were all aware of what was happening to me, since all the treatment was in the same hospital. I never expressed my frustration at the time, and, trying to be a good patient, I focused on getting through the ordeal.

The pre-op and post-op processes for my fourth surgery in July 2009 went much better. It was evident to me that the surgeon in charge had a great deal of influence on the amount of personal attention given to a patient, the choice of which floor/facility was assigned, and the ultimate well-being of the patient.

After this surgery, I was given a helmet—similar to a football helmet—to protect my head for the next six months. "I know I have to protect my head, but how can I wear this huge helmet at work?" I asked. "I need a better solution." A helpful nurse suggested I get a plastic insert and put it inside a baseball cap, so that it would be more comfortable.

August 2009 to February 2010

For the next six months, I wore the "hard" baseball cap throughout the day and removed it only to sleep and to take a shower. I was afraid of hitting my head getting in and out of the car or on a kitchen cabinet, for example. While it was not the most stylish headpiece, it eventually made for a lot of conversation and levity in the office.

The two years of health issues, however, took their toll on me, and I decided to accept an early retirement at the age of fifty-eight. Knowing that I had a fifth surgery ahead of me in 2010, and given the daily pressures of my job, I realized that taking care of my health was the main priority.

My last surgery occurred in February 2010. Worried the two back-to-back blizzards that winter might interfere with the planned surgery, my husband and I slept at a nearby hotel the night before so we could arrive by 5:30 a.m. Despite the unpredictability of the weather, the surgery did occur as planned, and by 12:30 p.m. I was in recovery. Remembering my last experience, I had asked my husband to please check on me periodically while I was in the recovery room.

There's a happy ending to the story, as after the fifth surgery, I fully recovered. I was fortunate I could advocate for myself throughout my experience, and, even after a surgical procedure, I could articulate my needs to the staff. But many other patients are not able to do so and are at the mercy of their healthcare providers and the system.

I wrote a letter to the president of the hospital describing my experiences. He contacted me and asked if I would participate on the newly formed Patient and Family Advisory Council (PFAC). I did and became the co-chair of the hospital PFAC and later co-chair of the entire hospital system's PFAC. Through our advisory council's input and involvement, we worked together to improve the hospital experience for other patients.

LESSONS LEARNED

The lessons learned from my healthcare experience provided the basis for many of the chapters in this book:

- When you are confronted with an unexpected illness, it is important to learn as much as possible about your condition, to be persistent, and to take charge of your health (Chapter 1).

- Two of the hardest tasks are to find and select the right physician (Chapter 3) and to decide where to go (Chapter 7). Reaching out to others can be an enormous help.

- Partnering with your doctor (Chapter 4) is critical. Asking questions and seeking a second opinion, if necessary, are vital to a successful outcome, particularly if a complication arises.

- The healthcare system can be terribly fragmented, especially when multiple practitioners are involved. The coordination of your care (Chapter 5) cannot be assumed to happen automatically and often is ultimately in your hands.

- A medical crisis can be an anxiety-filled experience. Finding ways to maintain your emotional well-being (Chapter 8) is just as important as treating your physical health.

- Sometimes, you may feel a healthcare practitioner doesn't fully understand what you are going through or is not taking you seriously. This could be due to biases and disparities in the healthcare system or to medical gaslighting (Chapter 10).

- When you are faced with a life-threatening condition, it is often difficult to talk about the end of life. However, being prepared in advance for the inevitable means you and your loved ones can focus on cherishing whatever time is left (Chapter 12).

COLETTE'S STORY

I knew from a very early age (seven or eight) that I wanted to be a doctor. Although my father was a physician, he never pushed me toward or away from medicine. When writing essays for medical school applications, my response to the question "Why do you want to be a doctor?" was typically "I love science, and I want to help people. Medicine will allow me to do both." That indeed was true and what I sincerely believed. It was a rational and logical reason to pursue a journey that required a tremendous investment of money (my parents'), time, effort, dedication, and stamina.

There was, however, so much more than that. I only became consciously aware of what that "much more" was about ten years ago. Age apparently has gifted me with the harvest of introspection and enabled me to gain insight internalized as a child but not understood at a conscious level back then.

When my sister and I were little, my father would sometimes take us to his office or on house calls. We would sit quietly in the waiting room, and I would watch as patients entered his office and exam rooms looking one way and then, later, emerge looking quite another. There was clearly something magical happening during that interaction. Furrowed brows, downcast eyes, or a cloak of fatigue were replaced by looks of relief, a sense of calm, or a stance of determination to fight whatever condition might be causing their physical or mental distress.

We would sit in the car as he went inside a stranger's home to care for someone for whom a visit to the office would prove a severe hardship or who could not afford a trip to the hospital. (Although there is renewed interest in doctors making house calls, and a few start-up companies currently provide primary care services in the home, at that time house calls were routine, particularly in small towns and rural areas.) Though he was sometimes paid not in money but in cakes, vegetables from a garden, and even the bounty of a recent hunting trip (I will never forget our kitchen sink with the frozen, skinned rabbit given to him by a patient—YUCK!), his passion, dedication, and joy in caring for his patients never flagged. Their lives were intertwined in a rare and special way.

As I look back on my training days in internship, residency, and fellowship, and later on my days in practice, certain moments are indelibly etched in my mind. I had the best role model in my father and received an excellent medical school education and training. And I have come to realize the fundamentals of quality, compassionate care, and stellar clinical outcomes remain the same.

These are but a few of those fundamentals born of the privilege I have had in caring for patients:

- Patients in a teaching hospital generally understand that some of their care will be provided by doctors in training. *As a medical student,* one evening I was sent to draw a blood gas test on a patient with asthma. A blood gas involves sticking a needle in a patient's wrist with the intent of drawing blood from an artery to determine how well the lungs are being oxygenated. Until the practice changed to injecting a little numbing medication prior to the blood gas needle stick, it was standard for this procedure to be performed without the benefit of anything to dull the pain. I always dreaded doing blood gases, because they could be difficult to perform and they were painful for the patient. After my third unsuccessful attempt, I told the patient I was going to get someone with more experience. She refused to let me do so, saying, "You have to learn. How are you going to learn if you don't keep practicing? You can do it, and I won't let anyone draw my blood but you." **You never know who your teacher will be.**

- *As a resident*, I learned the power of a gentle hand on a fevered brow, assuring a terminally ill patient you will be with them at the end and will make the journey as comfortable as possible, or saying "I'm so sorry" when someone is told the pregnancy test is negative after the fifth IVF (in vitro fertilization) cycle. I learned to look a patient directly in the eye and let him or her know, "I'll be with you every step of the way" as I deliver bad news, to stroke someone's hand until the pain medication kicks in, and to shower them with a sunshine-bright smile when the test for cancer comes back negative. **You never know when what is needed most is not the most cutting-edge technology or another blood test or a consult by the leader in the field, but being human and truly connecting with another person during a time of extreme vulnerability.**

- *As a GI (gastroenterology) fellow*, I was part of an on-call team presented with the challenge of providing care to a patient with a massive upper gastrointestinal bleed who was a Jehovah's Witness. Unfortunately, he had waited quite some time after he first began to bleed to tell his family he was having a problem. And then, once they were aware, much more time passed before they could convince him to go to the ER. He was quickly moved to the ICU and hooked up to IV fluids and medication to help stabilize him sufficiently for an endoscopy, which involved putting a scope with a camera down his esophagus to find out the source of the bleeding. He adamantly refused any blood transfusions. We discovered an ulcer in his stomach, which we treated, but we explained to him and his family that, given the amount of blood he had lost prior to coming to the hospital, he would die without being given (many) blood transfusions. In this literally life-and-death situation, his family, also of the Jehovah's Witness faith, attempted to convince him to accept the blood. With grace and an obvious love of his family and of life, he continued to refuse, and so we were left to keep him comfortable but helplessly watch as he slipped away. It was a devastating experience for his family, and what may be considered by some to be an unnecessary death haunted me. My sole source of comfort was the peace, faith, and equanimity with which he had accepted the consequences of the choices he had made, and seemingly without fear. **You never know when you will be called to remember that each moment with a patient is precious and should be honored as if it might be the last.**

- *As a physician in practice*, I was always surprised when a patient who had been seeking a diagnosis for quite some time before being referred to me would express shock and then relief when I said, "It doesn't make sense medically, and I can't explain it, but since you say it is happening, we need to move forward and figure out what is going on and what can be done about it. What do you think is going on? What do you think may be causing the problem?" Most of the time in these situations, the patient knew the puzzle pieces that led to the answer, and all we then needed to do in collaboration was to figure out how they fit together. **Never underestimate the power of stillness and actively listening in silence.**

In recounting these stories and thinking back on what has seemed to work in a one-on-one appointment with a patient, as well as at a large organizational systems level, I notice certain themes emerge. They may seem deceptively simple. Although everyone, both inside and outside the system, can rally and have an impact, translation into action at a population level requires passion, an unerring vision and belief in the possibility of a better and different way, and extreme perseverance.

So, as a healthcare provider, what works?

- **Do unto others as you would have them do unto you.** As you are interacting with patients (or with anyone, for that matter), imagine yourself in their position. Are you treating them in the manner you would want for yourself, a family member, or a friend? Do the staff and the design of the care delivery environment reflect an intention to bring ease to distress and suffering? Do your actions and words communicate best efforts and bring A-team performance to every encounter?

- **Focus on the patient.** If your focus remains on the patient and what is in their best interest, you will find there is greater clarity in decision-making and the actions you take (or select not to take because they really do not enhance your ability to diagnose, treat, or cure).

- **"*Sawubona*."** The translation from the Zulu is "I see you." Do your words and actions unequivocally let the patient know you see and respect them as a person with a real life, with real fears, and with ideas of their own about what may be wrong and what will work, or what may be best for them in addressing their medical issues? Do you communicate that you truly care and that you view the patient as not just a collection of signs, symptoms, and lab results to be "profiled" into a diagnostic bucket?

- **Be a healing presence.** Medicine is not nearly as black and white as we might think or like it to be. Despite all the awe-inspiring advances in technology, in medical techniques and interventions, and in lifesaving or life-changing medications, there is still a lot of gray area, and cure is not always possible. However, it is possible to heal even though you may not cure. Are patients left with a sense of peace, comfort, understanding, (reality-based) hope or optimism, and connection that engender (1) resilience and (2) the strength to move forward in the best direction for them, given their particular circumstances? Have they been helped to see and feel that their true essence remains intact, and that they are not merely their diagnoses?

These clinical lessons, combined with business school training and non-clinical professional experiences, influenced the selection of topics I thought were important to cover and those areas particularly thorny for patients to decipher and navigate.

The qualities I've described in the lessons that I learned in taking care of patients were those I provided to my patients. I believe they are also qualities that have become even more important in light of all the evolving advances in science, medicine, and technology.

In my opinion, at the end of the day, progress in those four areas should be complementary to and not a substitute for the relationships and trust between people that are critical to optimizing the health and well-being of patients. I think the qualities in my lessons learned are the qualities to which medical professionals aspire, and that can also make delivering care a more satisfying and less stressful experience for both providers and patients. Those behaviors help ensure that humanity is preserved as paramount in the midst of increasing opportunities to implement workflows and policies that are important to reducing the cost of care but that may sometimes be more focused on efficiency and on the system itself than on people.

Although it may not always feel that way, especially when we are sick, we all have more power than we realize, even as patients. This book also provides guidance regarding the many ways that power can be leveraged for the most important reasons of all—your health, well-being, and life itself and that of your loved ones.

It's "just" that "simple."

While there have been cutting-edge advances, innovative technologies, and new care delivery approaches, the lessons learned from the past can help take us "back to the future" in a way that brings insight, power, and grace to our patients as we face the myriad challenges of a complex healthcare system.

In a world of fragmented care, increasing complexity, a tsunami of chronic disease and lifestyle-related maladies, mounting healthcare costs, and a pandemic that has upended everyone's lives, caring and compassion remain paramount. It's just that simple.

LET'S START THE JOURNEY

As you can tell, both of us are very passionate about health, well-being, and the healthcare system. Much is needed to improve the quality and cost of care and to create a system that is easier to navigate and equitable for all.

The goal of this book is to provide guidance, insights, and practical tips that will help patients become empowered as they make their way through the challenges of the healthcare system. We hope it will provide the information, skills, and actions you can take to achieve optimal health and well-being for yourself and your loved ones, as well as arm you with tools to build the knowledge and self-confidence to advocate for the care you need and deserve!

CHAPTER 1

Taking Charge of Your Health

Doctors won't make you healthy. Nutritionists won't make you slim. Teachers won't make you smart. Gurus won't make you calm. Mentors won't make you rich. Trainers won't make you fit. Ultimately, you have to take responsibility. Save yourself.

NAVAL RAVIKANT

CHRIS' STORY

Chris was a career nurse, first at a community hospital and then working in the oncology unit of a multispecialty group practice. Working alongside many dedicated physicians, nurses, and staff, Chris had years of experience handling patients with difficult conditions and was well-versed in the operations of the healthcare system. However, it was her own unusual health issue that confounded her.

Chris was feeling fine until, at the age of forty-three, she noticed that her stomach would swell whenever she ate or drank. She had a complete gastrointestinal workup, but nothing was discovered. The distension progressed, and she began to vomit, even after two sips of water. She became very worried when her weight dropped from 120 pounds to 89 pounds. Because there was a family history of colon and prostate cancer—and she had survived a bout with breast cancer at age twenty-six—Chris decided to contact a cancer surgeon she knew and trusted at the hospital.

The surgeon performed some exploratory surgery but couldn't determine a diagnosis. He implanted a mediport under the skin to administer medications intravenously. In addition, a thin feeding tube was inserted from her nose to her small intestine for liquid nutrition.

Chris began to experience a high fever and chills. She had developed sepsis from the mediport, so the mediport had to be removed. Another one was inserted with extreme care, but another bout of sepsis ensued.

Chris began to develop allergies to the antibiotics. In response to her respiratory symptoms, she was given albuterol, a medication used to treat breathing problems and wheezing. The albuterol also caused an allergic reaction.

At one point, while Chris was in her hospital bed with a fever of 103 degrees, a young nurse began changing her IV bag. The nurse misread the instructions, and instead of 40 milligrams of Pepcid, she injected 40 units of insulin into the IV line. Although very tired and groggy, Chris caught the mistake in time, and the IV was turned off. *If I hadn't stopped her, I could have slipped into a coma and maybe even died*, Chris thought.

Her gastroenterologist emphasized the need to stay hydrated during this time and intravenously administered TPN (total parenteral nutrition), lifesaving nutrition for patients who cannot get nourishment orally.

Chris continued to undergo tests in the search to make a diagnosis. She went to an academic medical center in another state for motility tests to see if there was an abnormality in the movement of her GI tract. Even just eating toast and water continued to make her vomit. She was tested for a mitochondrial disease that affects the digestive system. The test was inconclusive.

After a CT scan, Chris was told she had spots on her pancreas. *Oh, no*, Chris thought, *I just can't win*. She called her cancer surgeon to review the scan. He responded, "I see nothing there. You're OK. Sometimes these get overread." Chris was relieved.

Without a clear diagnosis, Chris was then referred to a neurologist. He ran a battery of tests and discovered Chris had dysautonomia, a dysfunction of the nerves that regulate involuntary body functions such as heart rate, blood pressure, and sweating. Fortunately, he had a unique specialty in the dysfunction of the autonomic nervous system.

"Do you ever sweat?" the neurologist asked Chris.

"No, I never sweat," Chris replied. "I always hated the heat. I would feel like I was burning up inside whenever I would go to the beach. It never dawned on me this was a serious problem."

Chris also had very low blood pressure and a fixed heart rate. Sometimes her blood pressure was so low she could barely stand without feeling faint. Looking back on her life, she realized the dysautonomia was probably the root cause of many unusual conditions she had experienced.

Although Chris was glad to have a definitive diagnosis, she learned that, unfortunately, there was no cure for this condition. The symptoms come and go and must be treated as they occur.

So, Chris had to leave her nursing career and, with the support of her family, friends, and caring physicians, she continued to recover. "Sometimes I have to spend the entire day in bed because I'm so tired," Chris says, "but for the most part, I take it one day at a time. I don't push myself so hard any longer."

Chris continued to learn more about dysautonomia. "I am much better informed about this condition now," she commented. "I have discovered organizations that provide support and do research for this condition. Not all the information that I find online is reliable, so I have to determine what's real."

Throughout the entire ordeal, Chris kept copious notes. She maintained a written record of each test, procedure, medication, and dosage, as there was no other way to remember the details of her complicated medical history for each new doctor. She kept the name, address, and phone number of each physician she saw—including those of her pulmonologist, cardiologist, neurologist, surgeon, and endocrinologist. Her primary care physician was not able to manage this volume of detail, and Chris has had to coordinate her care herself.

She is grateful to those who have stood by her through the entire experience and continue to check in on her even now. Throughout this experience, Chris realized the importance of finding the right physician and the value of persistence, even when her condition seemed overwhelming. She especially appreciates the care of her neurologist, who has continued to follow her case throughout the years. She is also grateful for having a medical background herself, which enabled her to advocate assertively for herself as well as to manage at-home wound care, IV hydration, nutrition, and antibiotics, and to save herself on more than one occasion from avoidable, life-threatening situations while hospitalized.

LESSONS LEARNED

- Although Chris was a nurse and worked with many knowledgeable medical professionals, she was still challenged in finding answers to explain her condition. Chris' persistence and relentless search for the root cause of her illness proved to be the key to getting a diagnosis. Her presentation of symptoms did not fit into a "neat box" and was often different from what clinicians expected. Fortunately, she never gave up until the correct diagnosis was made and a treatment plan was implemented.

- Chris did her own research, asked questions, and kept detailed notes from every encounter with a medical practitioner. She took charge of her healthcare journey. Armed with knowledge, determination, and a willingness to communicate and coordinate care between her providers, Chris became the CEO (Chief Executive Officer) of her health and well-being.

WHAT YOU NEED TO KNOW

If you are struggling with a health condition and not sure what to do, here are some steps you can take to get started.

Pay Attention to Your Body

Taking charge of your health begins with first being aware of your own body, observing how it's functioning, and noticing any changes. Many of us take our health for granted when we are young, but as we age, we often notice that our bodies don't always respond the way we want. We'll talk more about ways to maintain good health in Chapter 2, but for now, take note of your current state.

Do you know your basic health measurements, such as your waist circumference, blood pressure, cholesterol, and blood glucose level? If elevated, they can be indicators or risk factors for heart disease, diabetes, and other chronic conditions, but many of us don't know what these numbers are and whether they're within the normal range.

While you don't want to become obsessive, take note of any physical changes such as changes in a mark or mole on the skin, or unusual lumps or growths. Have you recently gained or lost a lot of weight or noticed a change in your bowel habits?

Be aware of your psychological and emotional health as well. During the pandemic, many people experienced heightened anxiety and depression. An excessive amount of stress can affect you physically and mentally and impact your normal routine, as well as your sleeping, eating, and exercise habits.

Occasionally, there's a sense we don't quite feel right, but we ignore the signs and symptoms, hoping they will disappear or fearing the news will be bad. So, we put off going to the doctor, postpone our annual checkup or preventive care cancer screenings, and hope the problem will disappear on its own. Sometimes it does; however, you are the one who knows your body best, and when it sends signals, it is well worth paying attention.

Find a Primary Care Practitioner

Health is more than just the absence of disease; it's maintaining a state of well-being, both in mind and body. A key to taking charge of your health is to maintain regular checkups, customized to your specific situation, from a healthcare practitioner who knows your medical history, listens to your concerns, and coordinates your care when other specialists are involved. (See Chapter 3 for more information about the different types of healthcare providers who can function in this capacity.)

Do you have a primary care practitioner (PCP) who knows you well and can be contacted if necessary? The PCP will want to know your family history and complete medical history, including any past surgeries, injuries, and procedures as well as lifestyle habits. While your family history may not be the sole determinant of a particular condition, it may provide a clue to help with a diagnosis.

You will want to tell your physician about any allergies you have and describe the type of reaction, such as itching, rash, or difficulty breathing. You'll also want to provide a complete list of any medications you're taking—including the amount and frequency—as well as any vitamin supplements. Your primary care practitioner should recommend the screenings and vaccinations you need to maintain good health and provide any written orders if needed.

If you are experiencing a health problem and see your primary care practitioner, you will want to describe your symptoms in as much detail as possible. For example:

- How long have you been experiencing the symptoms, and how have they changed?

- Describe any pain or discomfort. Is it dull or acute, ongoing or sporadic? Is the area of the body tender to the touch?
- Do you feel any numbness or tingling? If so, where?
- Any dizziness or nausea?
- Any change in bowel habits?
- Any muscle cramps or spasms?
- Any unusual or excessive bleeding?

You will also want to convey your observations about any patterns in the symptoms. Does it seem to be worse at a particular time of day or night? Does it occur after you've eaten some particular food?

You'll also want to share any changes in your life that might be clues to explore. Has there been any change to your normal routine? Are you experiencing an unusual amount of personal or professional stress? Have you started or stopped any medication(s)?

While your healthcare practitioner will likely ask several questions, you may have an intuitive hunch about a possible cause of the problem and will want to share this observation. Could there be a prior injury or condition that is recurring? Although your information may not be relevant, sharing your thoughts might trigger action that could lead to the correct diagnosis. You know your body best, so trust your gut and convey as much information as you can.

Become More Health Literate

Even though you may not have a medical background, understanding basic medical terminology used in relation to your condition can help you communicate with your physician and contribute to the most appropriate treatment plan. While some of the information on the internet is not accurate or 100 percent reliable, it might be a place to start learning as much as possible about a particular health issue so you can ask the right questions. Being knowledgeable about your symptoms, possible causes, and treatment options can help you better understand and manage your care. Basic information about what medication is being prescribed, the dosage and frequency, and the possible side effects is important to taking it properly and to achieving the best outcome. If any adverse issues arise from the medication, you will want to communicate with your healthcare provider to see if changes to a regimen are warranted.

Ask for any literature and other resources available to help you better understand your condition. Don't be shy about saying "I don't understand" or "Can you explain what that means?" If there's a language barrier or limited cognitive ability, ask for someone to help explain the information, or bring along a friend or family member who can help translate, take notes, and clarify any instructions.

Do some research

Knowledge is indeed power; therefore, it is critical to ensure that you obtain knowledge from a credible source. In addition to the information you receive from your healthcare practitioners, you can also find a great amount on the internet. However, given the volume—as well as the growing amount of misinformation and sometimes outright scamming—it is important to identify sources that are well researched, that do not contradict scientific and medical facts, and that are intended to educate—not to convince you to buy a particular service or product.

Asking your healthcare practitioner for recommended websites is a good start. Below are some suggestions to help identify the many sources of credible information and to weed out the huge amount of misinformation now available at one's fingertips when you are searching on your own:

- Note the source of the information. Generally, websites such as ".gov" sites and those maintained by hospitals, academic institutions, and healthcare-related associations and nonpartisan foundations are reliable sources. Health and well-being sites—with editorial boards and evidence of recent and regular review by medical professionals—are generally considered to be reputable sources, although in some cases the information may not always be up to date.

- Pay attention to the website address.
  .gov = a government-sponsored site
  .edu = an educational institution
  .org = usually a noncommercial organization, but some have a specific agenda and mission that may bias the content
  .com = a business or commercial organization

- Be wary of sites that ask for your personal information or require payment to access them. Avoid sites that push products and services for which they receive a commission.

- Check to see if the site address starts with "https://" vs. "http://." Https sites are encrypted and less likely to be hacked.

- Check to see if the site provides a way to contact the host. It should also clearly state its terms and conditions of use.

Some safe sites that generally house accurate information include:

- MedlinePlus.gov—Sponsored by the National Library of Medicine [part of the National Institutes of Health (NIH)]
- MyHealthfinder at health.gov—Sponsored by the Office of Disease Prevention and Health Promotion in the U.S. Department of Health and Human Services (HHS)
- CDC.gov—Sponsored by the Center for Disease Control and Prevention
- NIH.gov—National Institutes of Health
- NIH List to Other Organizations (an NIH website page which lists all institutes within the NIH as well as other agencies pertinent to health and healthcare)
- FDA.gov—Sponsored by the Food and Drug Administration
- NCCIH.nih.gov—National Center for Complementary and Integrative Health (NCCIH)—The federal government's agency for scientific research on complementary and integrative health approaches
- PubMed® at Pubmed.ncbi.nlm.nih.gov—Contains information from scientific and medical journals

Know your health insurance benefits

Whether you obtain your health insurance through your employer or through a government-sponsored plan, it's important to know what's covered and what's not, to avoid any surprises and to help budget for medical expenses. When you enroll in an employer-sponsored health insurance plan, you should receive a summary plan description (SPD) outlining the coverage levels, the procedure to file a claim, and the appeal process. If you did not receive one, speak to your employer (or your company's human resource representative) or contact the appropriate government office. You are entitled to this information and shouldn't feel apologetic about asking for it.

Unfortunately, many people don't know the details of their health insurance plan until they receive a denial of a claim by the insurance company or a huge, unexpected bill.

Here's a quick self-assessment quiz to see if you can answer some basic questions about your healthcare coverage:

- What are the start and expiration dates? Is there a waiting period before the coverage begins? Does it end on the last day of employment or continue until the end of the month?

- Can you see any physician that you want, or do you have to seek care from a specified network? Are there different payments for in-network or out-of-network healthcare providers? How much do you have to pay for each?

- Do you need prior authorization for certain procedures or written referrals from a primary care practitioner before seeing a specialist?

- Are there any limitations or exclusions? For example, are you limited to a certain number of physical therapy treatments or chiropractic visits?

- Are certain procedures considered not medically necessary or experimental and not covered at all? How can you know for certain?

If you don't know the answers to these questions, contact the person in charge of your benefits at work or a customer service representative for your insurance company. If you are self-employed, your broker or applicable government agency can explain the coverage in your current health plan. Also, see Chapter 11 for a review of many common health insurance terms, such as deductibles, co-pays, and usual and prevailing rates.

Know your privacy rights

As a patient, you are entitled to the right of privacy of any information about your medical condition or treatment. Your privacy rights are protected under the federal law known as HIPAA (Health Insurance Portability and Accountability Act).

Whether the information is stored electronically or in a paper file, a healthcare practitioner cannot share this information with anyone unless specifically designated by you, whether to an employer, particular family member, or other patient (unless otherwise allowed by law). You can specify any individual with whom you do or do not want your information shared. You can also specify how you want to be contacted—for example, by email or phone—and note the contact information to be used as well as if a message can be left.

Under HIPAA, you have the right to see your medical records. If you see a mistake in the record or disagree with the notes, you have the right to get it corrected or send a written statement of the disagreement.

When you see a healthcare practitioner, you should be given a form outlining their compliance with HIPAA regulations. You will be asked to sign the form indicating your agreement or lack thereof with the terms. If you believe your privacy rights have been violated, consider first addressing the issue with your healthcare practitioner. If the matter cannot be resolved and the misuse of information has resulted in personal harm, you can file a complaint with the Office for Civil Rights at the U.S. Department of Health and Human Services.

Be Your Own Advocate
(and an Advocate for Your Loved Ones)

Taking charge of your health often requires persistence and perseverance. Medicine is both an art and an imperfect science. It is not as black-and-white as many might believe or hope it to be. Every patient is unique and may react to treatments differently. In addition, healthcare practitioners have varying levels of experience and expertise. Although they are very well educated, it is not possible for providers to know everything about every illness. They may be unfamiliar with certain medical conditions or symptoms and may need to refer you to a specialist. In some instances, several visits, tests, procedures, and different providers may be required to make a diagnosis, reach the correct conclusion about the underlying cause of a medical condition, or land on the appropriate treatment plan. Although it can be frustrating, don't give up!

You want to be an active participant in your care, not a passive recipient. Being your own advocate means partnering with your healthcare practitioner by discussing your condition openly, asking questions about treatment options, and determining the most appropriate next steps for you. (See Chapter 4.) You should be clear about what tests, procedures, and medications are being prescribed, what they are for, and any possible adverse effects that may occur. You also have the right to ask about the possibility of delaying action or choosing to follow a different course of action.

You have the right to be treated with respect by any healthcare professional, and if you feel you have not been listened to, or your care has not been managed properly, you should speak up in a politely assertive manner. As with the mix-up between potassium and insulin in Chris' story, you may have to act as your own advocate to prevent a serious or even deadly mistake.

Ask for Help

Taking charge of your own health at a time when you are feeling anxious, worried, and at your most vulnerable is not easy. Sometimes, even with our best efforts, we can't navigate the healthcare system successfully on our own. Asking for help from a family member, friend, or colleague who can act as your advocate can be invaluable. If that individual can accompany you on doctor visits, take notes, and ask questions on your behalf, you may have more clarity, better understanding, and more effective communication. It can be easy to forget instructions and next steps to take when you are back home, so having the detailed notes of a friend or family member can be very helpful.

You have the power to take charge of your health. Trust your instincts when something doesn't feel right, ask questions, learn as much as you can, and pursue the most appropriate care for you. Unfortunately, there are no guarantees, but at least you will know that you've done your best to achieve the most optimal outcome possible.

SO, WHAT CAN YOU DO NOW?

- Patients have more power than they realize and can use that power to take charge of their health and well-being. Although taking charge may seem daunting, the more you learn about how the system works, the rights you have, and the actions you can take, the easier it will be to advocate for yourself and your loved ones.

- Being proactive and seeking help from others can increase your chances of getting the care you need and deserve.

- Make sure you have a primary care practitioner (PCP).

- Be prepared for your medical and dental appointments. Make a list of any concerns. Be prepared to share any recent changes to your health, hospitalizations, and any changes to your prior medication regimen.

- Know as much as you can about your family history and the preventive care services you need, based on your age, sex, and personal/family history.

- Keep track of:
  - The medications you are taking, including OTC (over-the-counter), supplements, and herbal preparations, and why you are taking them. Ask about any potential side effects and harmful drug interactions that might be possible with your current medications.
  - Any allergies to medications, latex, immunizations, and preservatives, and the reaction you have to them.

- Your medical records, including copies of all lab results, x-rays, and pathology results. You may be able to download them if they are available through a patient portal.

CHAPTER 2

Embracing a Healthier Lifestyle

*If I'd known I was going to live this long,
I'd have taken better care of myself.*

EUBIE BLAKE

SUSAN'S STORY ABOUT RAY

It was May 2018, and Ray, age sixty-six, was planning to retire later that year. Working for a large international chemical company as a business development manager, Ray had already begun to delegate his responsibilities and train the individuals on his team. Going full steam until retirement, Ray had one last business trip to China, and then he could relax.

At six feet, five inches and 235 pounds, Ray was slightly overweight. He never smoked and rarely drank alcohol. However, at his last annual physical in 2016, the doctor said he had prediabetes and recommended he watch his diet carefully—and he had lost weight as a result of the modified diet. Because of his busy travel schedule, Ray skipped his 2017 physical. He figured he would schedule another one after he retired when he would have more time. Although he often felt tired, Ray attributed any fatigue to his demanding work schedule and travel. He submitted his retirement papers and, ignoring any physical symptoms, was determined to tough it out until he could finally leave his job.

The day before his China trip, Ray was mowing the lawn. His wife, Susan, found him in the garage, looking pale and sweaty. He was having chest pains and struggling to breathe. Suspecting a heart attack, she immediately took him to the community hospital nearby.

At the emergency room, they told him he may have had a mild "heart event." But a more immediate concern was a problem with his kidneys. Ray was put on an aspirin regimen for his heart and admitted to the hospital for further tests. Within a few days, the nephrologist ordered a kidney biopsy; however, because the aspirin regimen increased the risk of bleeding, the biopsy would have to wait a week. Ray's cardiologist wanted him to remain in the hospital during that time so they could closely monitor his heart function. Ray was put on statins to reduce his cholesterol.

A few days after Ray's discharge, his nephrologist called with the biopsy results. Ray had IgA nephropathy, an autoimmune kidney disease that occurs when an antibody builds up in the kidneys and the resulting inflammation hampers the ability of the kidneys to filter waste from the blood. Ray knew about his family history of IgA nephropathy but thought he had "dodged that bullet." The doctor prescribed a six-week course of the steroid prednisone beginning at 60 mg.

Back home from the hospital, Ray was feeling much better. With adjustments to his diet and careful monitoring of his blood pressure, Ray and Susan began to feel optimistic about managing the kidney disease and avoiding dialysis. But within a few weeks, a new problem arose. On June 11th, Ray's sixty-seventh birthday, Susan took him out to brunch and noticed that he was limping. A few days later, Ray complained of muscle aches and extreme fatigue. Ray then shared with Susan that a cut on the big toe of his right foot—a cut he had sustained earlier in the spring—hadn't healed and now looked infected. Susan looked at Ray's toe and was horrified. "It didn't even look like a toe anymore," Susan said. She reached out to a neighbor, a former ER nurse, who took one look at Ray's foot and said, "He needs to get to the hospital right now."

Ray had contracted MRSA (methicillin-resistant *Staphylococcus aureus*), a dangerous bacterial infection that can be difficult to treat. The orthopedic surgeon at the hospital advised that the best course of action was to amputate the toe.

During the surgery, Ray developed Afib, or atrial fibrillation, as his heart began to beat fast and irregularly. His cardiologist started him on Eliquis, a blood thinner, to prevent a stroke. Blood work showed that the infection had spread to Ray's bloodstream, so he was treated with the antibiotic vancomycin. After four days in the hospital with the antibiotic and blood thinner regimen, Ray began to feel better and was discharged. Upon discharge, his antibiotic was switched to daptomycin, and he continued to receive daily injections of the antibiotic on an outpatient basis for the next ten days.

By June 28th, Ray was cleared by the infectious disease doctors and was feeling great. Wearing a surgical boot, he was able to walk with a cane. The kidney disease had stabilized. And, at a visit with his cardiologist on July 3rd, he learned that his heart function had improved as well. Ray did mention that he was having some muscle aches and asked the cardiologist whether the statins he was taking could be the reason.

On Saturday, July 7th, he and Susan attended a wedding. During the reception, Ray wasn't feeling well, so they decided to leave early. Ray was so weak that he needed assistance to get to the car. He stayed in bed for the next day and a half. When the home health nurse came by to check his surgical wound on Monday, she noticed that his right leg was swollen. Even though Ray was taking a blood thinner, the nurse was concerned about a possible blood clot. She called Ray's internist, who ordered an ultrasound. Susan took Ray to the radiologist, but there was no clot. By the following day, July 10th, Ray was feeling very sick, and Susan took him back to the ER.

MRSA was still in Ray's bloodstream, and he had developed sepsis, a life-threatening complication of the infection. This time, Ray was given the antibiotic ceftaroline in addition to daptomycin to treat the MRSA. He remained hospitalized for three weeks.

Ray was very sick during the first week of this hospitalization. But even as he improved medically, and the MRSA finally cleared his bloodstream, he was increasingly discouraged and disheartened. Susan and Ray asked why he had been discharged from outpatient treatment in June if the MRSA infection was still in his body. The infectious disease specialists explained how insidious the MRSA bacteria can be. Ray's hemoglobin was low, and he received a blood transfusion. Ray's cardiologist and nephrologist followed him closely during his hospital stay.

Finally, on August 1st, Ray was ready to be discharged. The hospitalist suggested he spend time in a rehab facility before going home, but Ray refused. "The hospital feels like prison," he told Susan. "I just want to go home."

In anticipation of Ray's return home, Susan put a bed in the den on the first floor, where they also had a full bath. She arranged for home healthcare services and physical therapy, and she slept on the couch nearby. Their son built a wheelchair ramp in front of the house so Susan could more easily move Ray to the car for his doctor appointments.

Ray was elated and relieved to be back home. To continue the antibiotics, a central line port had been inserted so that Susan could give the daily infusions of daptomycin and ceftaroline. An infusion nurse came by once a week to change the dressing on Ray's port and to do a blood draw. A home health nurse came several times a week to change the dressing on the still-healing surgical wound on Ray's foot, and a physical therapist came to help Ray get moving again.

At a follow-up visit with the infectious disease doctor, the doctor advised that his liver enzymes in the first blood draw were at the high end of the normal range. Following the second week's blood draw, the doctor called Susan to say that his liver was failing. "You need to bring him into the ER," she said.

"No offense," Susan replied, "but we're going to a different hospital this time."

Susan helped Ray into the car and drove him to a large teaching hospital about ten miles from their home. There, he was diagnosed with an acute liver injury, likely caused by the ceftaroline. During this fourth hospital stay, Ray became pancytopenic, a condition in which the number of red and white blood cells, as well as platelets, is reduced. He developed lesions on his right leg, hip, and buttocks; these were ultimately diagnosed as ecthyma gangrenosum, a bacterial infection that typically occurs in patients who are critically ill and immunocompromised. His kidney status was also worsening. A scheduled liver biopsy was postponed as doctors worked to manage an increasing number of complex medical issues. At one point, Ray's blood pressure plummeted as his heart rate soared, and the rapid response team rushed in to stabilize him. He was transferred to the cardiac care unit.

The liver biopsy was finally performed on August 21st. On August 22nd, Ray was transferred by ambulance to a large, urban, teaching hospital in a neighboring state for evaluation of his liver failure and possible transplant evaluation.

Ray spent nine days in the ICU, where his liver function steadily improved. The MRSA was treated with vancomycin and the skin lesions with ciprofloxacin. He was started on intermittent dialysis for his renal failure. He didn't have much appetite, and the ICU doctor encouraged Susan to get him whatever he asked for—hamburgers, milkshakes—anything.

He was discharged from the ICU to a regular unit on August 31st and spent two more weeks in the hospital. Finally, on September 15th, Ray was discharged to the system's subacute rehab facility across the street. At rehab, Ray got stronger and, with assistance from a walker, was able to walk again. His kidney function improved, and he no longer needed dialysis. Mentally, he was upbeat and was looking forward to recovering at home. (A rehabilitation psychologist was an important part of the rehab team, and Ray benefited tremendously from the sessions with her.) Friends came for visits in the evenings and on weekends. Football season had started, and in the patient visitation area, Ray and Susan watched football games together.

An unexpected bonus was the rehab facility's excellent training for Susan on how to transfer Ray safely from the wheelchair to and from the car, his bed, and the toilet. "I was doing it all wrong," Susan realized. "They were wonderful."

"Should I get a chair lift for the house?" Susan asked the physical therapist.

"Not necessary," she replied. "With home physical therapy, he should be able to walk the stairs by Christmas."

So, on October 10th, Ray was discharged from the rehab facility and welcomed home by his family, friends, and members of his church community. Though still in a wheelchair, he no longer needed dialysis or infusions of antibiotics, but he was taking a number of medications, including coumadin (a blood thinner) for atrial fibrillation, midodrine for hypotension, Lasix (a diuretic), and ferrous sulfate (iron) for anemia. He was still taking prednisone, which had been prescribed for the IgA nephropathy; as a result, his blood sugar was occasionally high. Susan monitored his blood sugar with a glucose monitor and administered insulin as prescribed. Ray's appetite was good, and his strength continued to improve.

In mid-November, though, Ray developed a urinary tract infection (UTI), and Susan took him to the emergency room of a local hospital—one affiliated with the healthcare system from which he had been discharged most recently. The ER doctor prescribed another antibiotic. "I need you to consult with the downtown hospital," Susan said. They did. Happily, Ray did not need to be admitted.

With the UTI resolved, Ray was able to celebrate Thanksgiving at home. He went to his follow-up appointments every week and was getting physical therapy at home.

However, by the end of the first week of December, Ray appeared to have another UTI. He was lethargic and felt very ill. On December 9th, their son-in-law came over and helped Susan put him in the car. Ray didn't want to go all the way to the downtown hospital, so they opted for the teaching hospital about ten miles from home (the hospital where his liver injury was first treated back in August).

After a night in the ER while they waited for a room, Ray was admitted to the cardiac care unit. By the end of the week, he seemed to be improving but suddenly took a turn for the worse. His lungs had filled up with fluid, and he was incoherent, talking gibberish. The doctors sent Susan and her children home, telling her they planned to drain the fluid from Ray's lungs. The doctor called after the procedure and said his cognition had improved and he was resting comfortably. The next morning, Susan's phone rang. It was Ray calling from the phone in his hospital room.

"I came back to reality, and it's really a nice place to be," he joked. A few days later, he was moved to a step-down unit and continued making progress.

Christmas was approaching, and Ray was discharged to another rehab facility; unfortunately, he couldn't get a bed in the facility where he had made such great progress back in October. While the physical therapists at this new facility were good, Ray and Susan had concerns about the medication management. He seemed to be retaining a lot of fluid. After about a week, his improvement in physical therapy (PT) had plateaued. He seemed to grow weaker, not stronger. He was discharged in mid-January and seemed uncomfortable and lethargic, with no appetite.

At home, still on coumadin and several other medications, he gradually grew worse. He saw blood in his stools. Back to the hospital on February 2nd, doctors performed an endoscopy and discovered an ulcer. During the endoscopy, Ray became very unstable, and they moved him to the ICU for the next week until he stabilized and could be moved to the step-down unit once again. He was back on dialysis, and the nephrologist advised it would be permanent this time. Ray later told Susan how disappointed he was. The thrice-weekly dialysis would likely curtail all the fun trips they had planned for their retirement. "Maybe it will complicate travel abroad," she replied, "but there are dialysis centers all over the country. I'm sure we can figure it out."

On the following Monday, February 11th, Ray wished Susan a happy Valentine's Day.

It's not until Thursday, she thought. But she wished him a happy Valentine's Day, too. She was happy to see his appetite had returned.

By the following week, on February 19th, the doctors were talking about discharging him to rehab. Susan and Ray requested the downtown facility, and it seemed they might have a bed available. His cardiologists wanted to implant a subcutaneous defibrillator prior to discharge. Susan was optimistic.

Ray had his scheduled dialysis the following morning and called Susan at lunchtime when he was back in his room. A light snow was falling and was expected to continue through the evening. "Don't come over today," he said. "I don't want you driving home in the snow tonight." But two hours later, she received a call from the hospital. Ray had experienced "V-tach," or ventricular tachycardia, a problem with the heart's electrical impulses, and was transferred back to the cardiac care unit. After the stabilization of his heart, Ray remained in the CCU (cardiac care unit), where he received dialysis at the bedside several times. Doctors were concerned about his swallowing and prescribed a pureed diet that Ray found very unappealing. Even worse, his liquids had to be thickened, so he wasn't even drinking. Susan was alarmed and worried that he wasn't getting enough nourishment. *How can he possibly get better?* she thought. She asked Ray and the CCU doctor about a feeding tube, but Ray refused.

Susan stayed with Ray in the cardiac care unit all day Monday, but visitors (even family) had to leave the unit by 9:00 p.m., so she drove home. At 2:00 a.m., Susan received a call from the hospital. "Ray is having difficulty breathing," the nurse informed her. "We're going to intubate him."

"I'll be right there," Susan said. "Should I call my children?"

"Yes," the nurse replied.

When Susan arrived back at the hospital, the crisis had passed. Ray was sitting up in his bed with an oxygen mask on. He wanted to talk. "Something transformative is happening," he said.

"Ray was a very spiritual guy. He must have known he was dying," Susan said later, "but I didn't understand that at the time. I thought he had survived yet another crisis."

The nurse came in and told Susan not to let Ray take his mask off to talk, so the conversation ended. She stayed by his side for the next few hours while he dozed.

At 6:30 a.m., the nurse told Susan she had to leave the unit and that she could return at 11:00 a.m. when normal visiting hours resumed. "Should I stay in the waiting area?" Susan asked the nurse.

"He's stable now," he replied. "Go home and get some rest."

Susan called the kids and told them their dad was stable. Their son, who lived several hours away, planned to take a train later that morning and would arrive by noon. Their daughter, a teacher who lived nearby, planned to get a substitute for the afternoon.

Susan went home to take a shower and the phone rang again. It was the hospital. She dressed quickly and arrived at the CCU with her friend, the retired ER nurse. As they stood in the hall talking to the CCU doctor, Ray gave Susan a little wave. It was the last time she saw him conscious.

The doctor told Susan that Ray's organs were failing. He explained that, in addition to administering various medications intravenously to keep his blood pressure up, they'd have to intubate him to keep him alive. And even then, it would only sustain him for a few more hours. "Or we can allow him to pass peacefully now," he said.

Susan was stunned. "She wants her children to get here," her friend said.

Their son and daughter arrived, along with their minister and two of Ray's sisters. (Ray had been sedated prior to intubation, so he wasn't conscious.) The family spent the afternoon and early evening by his side, telling him how much they loved him. Around 6:00 p.m., the nurse came in to say that one of the IV medications was about to run out; he could hang another bag, he said, but the family agreed that Ray had been through enough. Ray passed at 6:14 p.m.

In retrospect, Susan wished that she and Ray had paid more attention to his health and had been more proactive. Perhaps if he hadn't put off his annual physical in 2017, he might have detected his kidney disease earlier, before it had advanced to stage 4. If they had focused on his prediabetic condition, the wound on his foot might have healed more quickly, and he could have avoided the MRSA infection. Susan thought perhaps this whole calamitous chain of events could have been avoided, and Ray might still be alive today.

LESSONS LEARNED

- Ray's tragic story is a wake-up call exemplifying the importance of being proactive and taking prevention seriously. With busy lives, many people may delay routine visits with their primary care practitioner and may not follow through with preventive care. That means lost opportunities to detect issues early, to get immunizations and screenings to avoid problems altogether, and to lessen the impact of preexisting conditions.

- Ignoring early signs of disease and putting off seeking medical attention can be the difference between life, avoidable disability, and premature death.

- Many of the most prevalent conditions in the U.S. are lifestyle related. Heart disease, for example, could potentially be prevented through actions we can take—eating a healthy diet, managing stress, getting sleep of good quality and sufficient duration, and not using tobacco or vaping products. Maintaining a healthy lifestyle can make a big difference in both the quality and longevity of our lives.

WHAT YOU NEED TO KNOW

Perhaps if Ray had followed up with his primary care physician as requested, the doctor could have become more involved in his care, and maybe the ensuing events could have turned out differently.

Get a PCP

As mentioned in Chapter 1, having a primary care practitioner (PCP) who can monitor and coordinate your care is a good first step. An effective PCP, one who knows you and your medical history, can provide continuity of care and coordination when multiple specialists are involved. In addition to providing checkups based on age, sex, and medical history, PCPs can advise you of the recommended immunizations, like flu and pneumonia vaccines; cancer screenings, such as mammograms and colonoscopies; as well as any follow-up and subsequent care.

SOME CANCER SCREENINGS[1]

The lifetime risk for invasive cancer is one in two for men and one in three for women, so early detection is key to survival. Moreover, the risk of most cancers increases as you get older. Consult with your healthcare practitioner about the timing and type of screening options, depending on such factors as your age and sex, as well as your personal and family medical history. Often there are no warning signs, which makes early detection critically important. However, any signs or symptoms of the disease that do appear should prompt a discussion with your healthcare practitioner regarding next steps.

Type of Cancer	Who Should Get Screened?	Screening	Some Possible Signs & Symptoms
Breast	Women High-risk men[2]: age over fifty with family history of breast cancer, genetic mutations, radiation therapy to the chest, hormone therapy, liver disease, obesity	Mammogram MRI (magnetic resonance imaging) Ultrasound	Lump in breast/underarm Change in size/shape of breast Discharge from nipple
Cervical	Women Transgender: female to male with cervix intact	Pap smear HPV (human papillomavirus) test	Heavy bleeding Pelvic pain
Colorectal	Men & women	Colonoscopy Blood-based test Stool-based test (e.g., Cologuard)	Blood in stool Persistent change in bowel habits Abdominal discomfort Unexplained weight loss
Lung	Men & women	Low-dose CT scan	History of smoking Persistent cough Shortness of breath
Melanoma/Skin	Men & women	Total body skin check	Change in size/shape/color of mole New/unusual growth Sore that doesn't heal
Oral	Men & women	Visual X-ray	Sore, lump, or ulcer in the mouth that doesn't heal
Prostate	Men Transgender: male to female	PSA blood test (prostate-specific antigen) Digital exam	Trouble urinating Blood in urine/semen

Note: These are just a few of the cancer screenings that are available. Guidelines are updated regularly, so be sure to talk with your healthcare practitioner to determine what might be right for you based on your particular situation. For more information, see the Resources section at the back of the book.

Your PCP can also keep you up to date on the immunizations needed for your age, sex, and personal history, such as those to prevent the flu, shingles, pneumonia, and other viral or bacterial related conditions. The COVID-19 vaccine, along with boosters, has been added to the list and has proven to be the best way to prevent serious illness, hospitalization, and death from the virus.

Unfortunately, at least 25 percent of individuals in the U.S. do not have a PCP—and that percentage is growing. It's even worse for younger Americans: only 64 percent of Americans in their thirties have one. In some cases, individuals have used urgent care centers and walk-in clinics instead of having a PCP, but these centers do not monitor a person's care over time and are not set up to provide primary care services.

People who see their PCPs consistently have been found to have better health outcomes with lower costs.[3] Although there has been a recent upsurge in the number of medical school applications and primary care specialties,[4] a physician shortage exists and has been further exacerbated by the pandemic. And with an aging population, the demand for primary care is growing. Nurse practitioners (NPs) and physician assistants/associates (PAs) are often more commonly filling this role in many places.[5] Finding the right healthcare practitioner—someone you trust and who can offer the services you need—is critical to prevention.

See Your Dentist

In addition to a PCP, it's important to have a dentist who can monitor your oral health. Some people are not aware that the bacteria and inflammation caused by tooth decay and periodontal (gum) disease can lead to health problems throughout the entire body. Aching teeth, bad breath, and bleeding gums (symptoms of periodontal disease) can increase the risk of cardiovascular disease, including heart attacks and strokes, as well as premature delivery in pregnant women. It can make diabetes more difficult to manage. Additionally, poor oral health may contribute to dementia, respiratory infections, pregnancy complications, infertility, erectile dysfunction, rheumatoid arthritis, cancer, and kidney disease.[6] Prevention is the key. Proper daily dental hygiene—brushing and flossing—and regular, twice-a-year visits to the dentist can help prevent more serious health issues.

The Importance of a Healthy Lifestyle

During the COVID-19 pandemic, individuals with underlying chronic illnesses have been among the most vulnerable. Of the over one million Americans who have died during the pandemic to date, many were already suffering from heart disease, cancer, and diabetes, the leading causes of death and disability in the U.S. These underlying chronic diseases, along with a weakened immune system and other conditions, posed a greater risk of severe complications, hospitalization, and death from COVID-19. And those most severely impacted were communities of color, people in rural areas, and those of lower socioeconomic status, all groups that carry a heavier chronic disease burden.

According to the CDC (Centers for Disease Control and Prevention), chronic and mental health conditions account for 90 percent of the $4.1 trillion spent annually on healthcare in the U.S.,[7] the highest of any country in the world,[8] and this number continues to grow. However, while genetics do play a role in certain individuals, many chronic health conditions can be prevented, or at least mitigated, by making changes to our lifestyle.

Smoking, unhealthy eating, lack of physical activity, poor quality sleep of insufficient duration, high levels of stress, and a low degree of connection and sense of community have been shown to be the most detrimental factors influencing our health, well-being, and longevity. If you can take even small steps to improve your lifestyle habits, and strengthen your immune system at the same time, perhaps you can avoid succumbing to these disabling conditions or at least mitigate their negative consequences.

While much has been written about maintaining a healthy lifestyle, here are some basic reminders to minimize the risk of developing a chronic disease and/or cancer and boosting your natural immunity as well.

Quit smoking

Cigarette smoking has fallen to an all-time low in the U.S., thanks to public health warnings, increased taxes on tobacco products, and smoking bans in many states. Yet, according to the CDC, nearly forty million adults still smoke cigarettes. Adding in e-cigarettes and other forms of tobacco (e.g., cigars and chewing tobacco), there are about forty-seven million users, or 19.3 percent of the adult population. In addition, about 4.7 million middle- and high-school students use at least one tobacco product.[9]

Nearly 70 percent of smokers say they want to quit, but nicotine addiction is strong. The CDC says, on average, it takes eight to eleven attempts to quit. Other research puts the number as high as thirty attempts. The "cold turkey" method is the least successful, as only 3–5 percent quit for longer than six months. A combination of counseling and medications has a much higher success rate. Most importantly, if a doctor discusses tobacco use and the need to quit, a patient is twice as likely to stop. And support from family and friends increases the likelihood of being successful.

The short- and long-term benefits of quitting smoking to your health are noteworthy.[10] Within one to nine months of quitting, lungs continue to improve and heal, reducing coughing and shortness of breath. Within five years, the risk of mouth, throat, esophagus, and bladder cancer decreases by half; cervical cancer and stroke risks decline to the level of a non-smoker. So, the sooner you quit, the sooner you can reap the benefits to your health.

Eat wisely

One of the most important ways to prevent disease is to improve what we eat.[11] Our addiction to sugary drinks and highly processed foods has led to a huge increase in the obesity rate. According to a 2020 CDC report, 42 percent of those living in the U.S. are obese. Besides increasing the risk of diabetes, heart disease, stroke, and cancer, medical costs for those with obesity are close to $1,900 higher each year than for people who are at a healthy weight.[12] We have an important choice to make, every day. According to Dr. Mark Hyman in his book, *Food Fix*, our food can serve as medicine for our bodies or as an agent of disease.

Research has shown that the health of the microbiome—the number and diversity of microorganisms like bacteria and fungi in our gut—is key to our well-being. The health of our gastrointestinal system has been linked to our body's immune system, and problems in the gut can be the cause of chronic inflammation leading to the chronic conditions mentioned earlier.[13]

Unfortunately, most clinicians have never been trained in nutrition, as it typically has not been part of the medical/nursing/pharmacy school curriculum in the past. And, unless a clinician has a keen interest in additional learning, the likelihood of gaining a sufficient knowledge base to counsel patients effectively is low. Individuals may need to seek the help of someone trained in nutrition (e.g., a registered dietitian) or a functional medicine specialist to advise on healthy eating practices.

While there are many weight-loss programs and fad diets marketed in the U.S., numerous studies have found the Mediterranean diet to be the best to reduce the risk for diabetes, heart disease, and cancer. It has also been shown to benefit brain health, including reducing the risk of dementia, memory loss, and depression.

The Mediterranean diet[14] is rich in plant-based foods, including fruits, vegetables, whole grains, legumes, and nuts. The emphasis is on healthy fats—extra virgin olive oil (instead of butter and margarine), avocados, nuts, and oily fish, like salmon and sardines.

Much smaller amounts of other sources of protein, such as poultry, dairy, and eggs are eaten. Red meat consumption is minimal and limited to twice per month. Water is the main beverage, but a moderate amount of red wine is allowed.

Much has been written about eating organic foods, free of pesticides, as well as non-genetically modified (non-GMO) vegetables and fruit, and antibiotic- and hormone-free meats. We have been told to increase our fiber with more fruits and vegetables and to drink more water. But why haven't we been successful?

- Like smoking, the addiction to sugar and processed food can be overwhelming. Our cravings are powerful, and deep-seated eating habits are conditioned early on from childhood.

- Fresh produce, non-GMO products, antibiotic- and hormone-free meats, and organic food are more expensive and less readily available in some areas. They may be impossible to find in "food deserts" (areas with little access to affordable, nutritious food) and "food swamps" (areas with a predominance of high-calorie, junk-food establishments). Yes, organic foods are more expensive, but so are our healthcare costs.

- While the connection between smoking, alcohol, and cancer has been well established as a public health issue,

GUIDELINES FOR DRINKING IN MODERATION[16]

1 Drink or Less per Day for Women

2 Drinks or Less per Day for Men

Standard Drink Sizes for One Drink
(ABV=alcohol by volume):
- 12 ounces of beer (5 percent ABV)
- 8 ounces of malt liquor (7 percent ABV)
- 5 ounces of wine (12 percent ABV)
- 1.5 ounces of 40 percent ABV (80 proof) distilled spirits (gin, rum, vodka, whiskey, etc.)

the correlation between our food supply and our health has not been widely endorsed or sufficiently communicated. The power of the food industry and associated lobbyists and associations is great and makes any nationwide changes in our eating patterns a daunting challenge. However, even given this reality, companies have been pushed by the public to provide healthier options as well as production with a lower carbon footprint.

The journey to better health and well-being is a personal one, and we must make our own decisions about what to eat and how to adjust our eating habits. Small incremental changes are usually best, and there are wonderful resources to help. For now, the mantra of Michael Pollan in his book *In Defense of Food: An Eater's Manifesto* is good to remember: "Eat [real] food. Not too much. Mostly plants."

Be judicious about alcohol

There is currently no consensus within the medical community regarding alcohol. While some believe intake in moderation may provide benefits, some studies suggest there is no safe amount of alcohol because of the link to an increased risk of cancer[15] (breast, colon, liver in those who develop cirrhosis, head and neck, and esophagus). Excessive alcohol can also play a role in the development of high blood pressure, heart disease, GI (gastrointestinal) problems, dementia, stroke, liver disease, depression, and alcohol use disorder.

Keep moving

You've also heard a great deal about the benefits of physical activity. Regular physical activity, along with healthy eating, is important to managing one's weight and preventing obesity. Aerobic exercise, along with resistance training, can maximize fat loss and maintain muscle, which are both essential for optimal metabolism.

TIPS TO GET MOVING

- Take the stairs instead of the elevator.
- Park a little farther away than normal from the entrance at your destination.
- Take a walk.
- If you spend much of the day sitting, get up and stretch every thirty to sixty minutes.
- Find a friend to work out with. When someone is waiting, you are more apt to keep the appointment.
- If you use a treadmill or stationary bike at home or at a gym, listen to music or watch a movie while you're exercising.
- Make it a family affair, so you can talk and spend time together while you're physically active.
- Join a class or walking club to make it a regular social event.
- If you can afford it, find a trainer to help you get started. Some gyms include a consultation as a benefit of membership, and virtual options may also be available.
- There are many free online videos that can be selected based on your goals, your fitness level, and degree and type of mobility.

In addition to helping us reach and maintain a healthy weight, regular physical activity can reduce the risk of a heart-related illness by improving circulation and lowering blood pressure. Exercise can lower blood-sugar levels and can help reduce the risk of type 2 diabetes. Regular physical movement has also been shown to reduce the risk of some cancers, including colon, breast, uterine, and lung cancer. Moreover, balance and muscle-building exercises can reduce the risk of falls—and subsequent hip fractures—and weight-bearing exercise plays an important role in combating osteoporosis as we age.

During exercise, chemicals called endorphins are released; they trigger a positive feeling in the body and can improve your mood and help you deal with stress. Physical activity also stimulates the release of dopamine, norepinephrine, and serotonin that are important to regulating your mood. Studies have shown that physical activity can be as effective as medication in some individuals suffering from mild to moderate depression![17]

For those who may have limited mobility—perhaps due to multiple sclerosis (MS) or Parkinson's—and experience balance issues or are confined to a wheelchair, there are still ways to engage. For example, exercises specifically designed to improve balance can be performed in a seated position. Many online exercise videos labeled for seniors have applicability to everyone. And a physical therapist, experienced in the care of people with neuromuscular disorders, can help design a program of physical activity specific to a patient's symptoms.

With the demanding pressures of our daily lives, what can we do to make physical activity a part of our daily routine? You don't have to run a marathon, join a gym, or play a competitive sport. As with all other lifestyle changes, starting small can make things easier, and engaging in physical activity that you enjoy means you are more likely to be consistent and participate regularly.

Recent studies have indicated that every little bit helps. Even a few minutes per day of light-to-moderate physical activity was associated with significantly lower risks of premature death.[18]

Of course, consult your healthcare practitioner first to map out the best plan for you. If you experience chest pain, severe shortness of breath, or other symptoms you have not previously felt before, stop immediately and check with your physician.

Get enough high-quality sleep

Sleep is essential to our overall health and well-being, yet many people get less than the recommended seven to eight hours of sleep per night. According to the CDC, 35 percent of adults in the U.S. do not get seven hours of sleep per day.[19]

In addition, 48 percent of people in the U.S. report snoring problems, according to the CDC. And twenty-five million U.S. adults suffer from obstructive sleep apnea, which is more prevalent in men.[20]

As we age, it's not that we need more sleep, but we tend to have a harder time falling asleep and more trouble staying asleep than when we were younger. People over the age of sixty are more likely to experience sleep problems from a variety of health conditions, such as reflux (heartburn), pain from osteoarthritis, trips to the bathroom in the middle of the night due to enlarged prostate or overactive bladder, and depression and anxiety. And some sleep problems can be attributed to the medications used to treat these conditions.

TIPS FOR GETTING A GOOD NIGHT'S SLEEP

- Maintain a regular sleep schedule, going to bed and waking at the same time each day, even on weekends.

- Adopt a pre-bedtime routine during which you wind down and de-stress, signaling the body it's time to sleep.

- Avoid electronics (e.g., smartphones, computer, TV, etc.) before bedtime to minimize the blue-light exposure and stimulation.

- Keep the bedroom dark and cool (60 to 67 degrees).

- Avoid alcohol and heavy meals later in the evening. Alcohol may help you fall asleep more easily but can be disruptive and lead to poor quality sleep during the night. Eating too late can cause digestive issues such as reflux that may impact sleep.

- Include some regular physical activity in your daily routine but avoid rigorous exercise late in the evening or in the two to four hours before you go to bed.

- Update your mattress if it's worn out and uncomfortable.

- Discuss supplements, like melatonin, with your PCP. Though helpful to some, melatonin doesn't work for everyone. It is important to use the proper dose; more is not better. In fact, for some people, it can actually worsen sleep problems and should be avoided altogether.

Why is sleep so important to our health? Sleep is the time when our body heals itself; it repairs the damage to our cells from stress and from harmful exposures. Better sleep helps our body fight infection by boosting our immune system. Sleep also provides a "housekeeping" role that removes toxins that build up in our brains when we're awake. Research is indicating this cleansing of the brain can help reduce the risk of Alzheimer's disease and other dementias.

Lack of sleep has been associated with a greater risk of heart disease and stroke, as it affects blood pressure and cholesterol levels. Poor sleep also has adverse effects on blood sugar levels, with a strong link to type 2 diabetes. It increases our stress hormones, which affects the level of inflammation in our body—a risk factor for cardiovascular conditions like heart disease and stroke.

Sleep also affects our ability to lose weight. The hormones ghrelin, which stimulates appetite, and leptin, which suppresses appetite, are impacted by a lack of sleep. Good sleepers tend to eat fewer calories.[21]

Mental health is impacted as well. Ninety percent of people with depression complain about sleep quality. Lack of sleep disrupts the body's levels of the hormones—including serotonin, dopamine, and cortisol—that affect thought, mood, and energy. People with serotonin deficiencies are more likely to suffer from depression.[22]

If sleep problems persist, and you're constantly exhausted, you may be putting your health and safety at risk as well as that of others. Many car accidents occur when drivers are sleepy at the wheel. Those who work a night shift may also experience sleep problems, such as insomnia and excessive sleepiness, that can impact their health and lead to mistakes and accidents.[23] It's wise to see a professional sleep expert to diagnose the underlying cause and find ways to overcome sleep issues.

Manage your stress and build resilience

We all have stress in our lives. Work demands, family issues, rush-hour traffic, financial worries, fears of catching a contagious virus—all create mounting stress that can take a toll on our health and well-being. While we will not be able to eliminate all these stressors in our lives, we may be able to find ways to manage our response to them.

Our reaction to stress can include headaches, muscle tension, fatigue, stomach upset, sleep problems, and much more. If it continues unmanaged, stress can lead to burnout and chronic diseases, including high blood pressure, heart disease, diabetes, and obesity.

The recent coronavirus pandemic, along with physical isolation, created a heightened sense of anxiety and stress for many individuals. It negatively impacted many of our lifestyle behaviors, including our daily eating habits, the amount of regular physical activity, and our normal sleep patterns. A proliferation of stress-relieving methods emerged during these difficult times, including meditation apps that can be downloaded to a smartphone, virtual exercise classes, and online cognitive behavioral therapy (CBT).

Each person can find his or her own way of handling life's stressors, as there's no one-size-fits-all solution. However, if a high level of stress persists, it's important to seek the help of a mental health professional.

In studies regarding human longevity, other factors—in addition to healthy eating, physical activity, adequate sleep, stress reduction, and not smoking—affect how people can not only live longer but also maintain the quality of their health and well-being for a longer period of time. Dan Buettner, in his book *The Blue Zones*, researched the areas in the world in which an inordinate number of people live to the age of one hundred and beyond. Their lifestyles include a strong sense of community, and the quality of their relationships helps provide support. There's also spirituality among the people—not necessarily in a religious sense—that includes an appreciation of nature and a gratitude for life.

These individuals, who may work well into their nineties, have a sense of purpose and meaning in their lives. While they may not have the most money or access to the latest medical and technological advances, the people in these

SOME WAYS TO REDUCE STRESS

- Deep breathing and meditation
- Practicing mindfulness
- Using guided imagery
- Establishing a gratitude practice
- Practicing yoga, yoga nidra, or tai chi
- Laughing
- Spending time with family and friends
- Spending time in nature
- Turning off the social media
- Spending time on a hobby—gardening, art, music, reading, etc.
- Volunteering to help others
- Talking to a coach or counselor

communities have shown how everyday lifestyle, human connection, and purpose can prevent many of the chronic diseases that plague so many others around the world.

Our healthcare system is designed to treat disease, with not enough focus on prevention. It cannot ensure that everyone stays well. So, the responsibility for maintaining your health and well-being is ultimately up to you. While we can't control everything in our environment, we can strive to take control of our lifestyle habits and avoid many preventable chronic diseases. Start now. Your health is in your hands!

SO, WHAT CAN YOU DO NOW?

- Eighty percent of the conditions responsible for the greatest burden in healthcare in the U.S. are potentially preventable. You have the power to positively impact your physical and mental health and well-being. Prevention is still the best medicine!

- Living a healthy lifestyle—including not smoking, healthy eating, regular physical activity, sleep of sufficient duration and quality, managing stress, moderate alcohol use (if at all), and living in community with connections to others—is a powerful way to increase your longevity, reduce the risk of chronic conditions and cancer, and mitigate their impact if they develop.

- Find a medical practitioner with whom you have a collaborative, trusting relationship in which you feel heard and respected.

- Request a consultation with a registered dietitian to ensure you know how to eat in a healthy way based on your personal and family medical history, your culture, and your budget. And get guidance from your healthcare practitioner regarding a regular routine of physical activity.

- Make sure you know the cancer screenings you need based on your age, sex, and personal and family history.

CHAPTER 3

Choosing the Type of Doctor You Need

I think the extreme complexity of medicine has become more than an individual clinician can handle. But not more than teams of clinicians can handle.

ATUL GAWANDE, MD

MARGARET'S STORY ABOUT ROBERT

In 1966, when Robert was eighteen years old, he was diagnosed with Hodgkin's disease and treated with heavy doses of radiation, which was the most effective treatment at that time. Eventually cured, Robert went on to lead a healthy life with his wife, Margaret. However, in 2014, at age sixty-six, he began to retain fluid in his body, experienced shortness of breath, and grew anxious. An avid golfer, Robert was suddenly afraid to play a round of golf with his friends.

With guidance from his niece, a physician, he made an appointment—after a two-month wait—with a well-known cardiologist at a large teaching hospital. Robert learned his case was unusual; the radiation he received as a teenager had calcified his arteries and the pericardium, which surrounds the heart, might have to be surgically removed. Many of the younger doctors had never seen this condition before, as the high-dose radiation regimen to treat Hodgkin's disease had changed many years ago. Robert's doctor stated, "You are the last man standing with this condition."

Robert was treated with a high dose of steroids. And to address his anxiety, Robert was seen by a psychologist at the same hospital. While he was at the hospital, a surgeon and a hematologist were also consulted.

An internal medicine physician assigned to Robert's case acted as the "quarterback" to coordinate the four, and sometimes five, doctors who would meet with Robert and Margaret. The team of physicians met every morning during the week to discuss the patients who were under their care. They would review Robert's latest blood work results, the scheduled tests, and the various treatment options that were suggested. Later in the morning, the lead physician would relay the team's deliberations and the group's decisions to Robert and Margaret.

These team meetings proved to be critically important to Robert's care. For example, one physician suggested that Robert be given a diuretic to reduce the fluid buildup in his body. "No, no, no," the cardiologist immediately interjected. "He's on this medication, and, if given that diuretic, he could go into renal failure." The cardiologist, at that moment, was in Canada and had phoned into the meeting.

After three weeks, Robert left the hospital and returned home. He began seeing his local cardiologist every three months to do further tests, and he continued to improve for the next two years. He was back playing golf regularly and continuing his consulting business.

Margaret, who had always accompanied Robert to all his doctor visits, kept a journal of every conversation and interaction. She never hesitated to ask a question to clarify a specific term or procedure. Often on the way home, Robert would comment about what he thought the doctor had advised. Occasionally, Margaret would have to refer to the notes in her journal to clarify the doctor's orders. For example, Robert thought the cardiologist had recommended he wear compression socks 24/7; however, the notes indicated the doctor suggested not wearing the compression socks while sleeping.

In 2016, Robert began to lose weight, and by the winter, he returned to the teaching hospital. His aortic valve had further calcified. There was a discussion about whether he would need a type of surgery called TAVR (transcatheter aortic valve replacement), which is a minimally invasive procedure to replace a narrowed aortic valve that fails to open properly (aortic valve stenosis). TAVR surgery was successfully performed in December 2016.

In 2017, Robert and Margaret decided to move to Florida to be closer to Robert's family. They rented an apartment while their new house was being built, and in March 2018, they settled into their new home.

Seven weeks later, however, Robert suddenly became ill. He was vomiting, becoming dehydrated, and rapidly losing weight. Margaret took him to the local emergency room to figure out what was wrong. The gastroenterologist, assuming this was an intestinal flu bug, quickly put him on an IV to restore his fluids and admitted him to the hospital. The vomiting continued, and numerous tests were inconclusive.

After three days in the local hospital, Margaret contacted Robert's niece, the physician who was knowledgeable about Robert's medical history. She recommended that Margaret get Robert to the hospital where she practiced, the same location as Robert's regular cardiologist.

After a review of Robert's previous tests and his medical history, the gastroenterologist assigned to Robert's case suggested a biopsy of his bile ducts. She discovered that Robert had cholangiocarcinoma, a rare cancer of the bile ducts. The team suggested chemotherapy treatment. However, after two rounds of chemo, it was determined the chemo treatment was not effective. The palliative care team visited with Robert and Margaret to discuss hospice.

"What will happen to him?" Margaret asked Robert's niece. "What can I expect?"

His niece provided Margaret with the information she needed, "Robert will continue to get weaker, and eventually, his body will shut down." By November 2018, just a few weeks shy of his seventieth birthday, Robert died.

The intense radiation Robert received as a teenager had taken its toll, slowly compromising his body and internal organs. Nevertheless, Margaret was appreciative of the excellent, coordinated care he received at the teaching hospital. The right doctors, working as a team, and the right hospital had made a significant impact on the quality of life that Robert enjoyed during the last few years of his life.

LESSONS LEARNED

- Margaret and Robert sought the care of a variety of medical specialists to treat Robert's illnesses. With each new condition, they were fortunate to have a doctor and two nurses in the family who could help with questions to ask and help manage expectations. While many people will not have a medical professional in the family, reaching out to others for information and referrals can prove to be helpful.

- Although Robert finally succumbed to cancer, the doctors worked as a team to manage Robert's care. This team approach helped coordinate Robert's treatment and avoid potential errors.

- Margaret played a critical role as Robert's advocate by taking notes, asking questions, and providing support throughout his healthcare journey.

WHAT YOU NEED TO KNOW

For most of us, getting to the right healthcare provider may be a matter of chance or a process of trial and error. Because clinicians may be on different electronic medical record systems or have no means to ensure everyone receives a copy of the documentation from the various care settings a patient may access, many medical providers are often unaware of the treatment being rendered by others.

Knowing the role of the various types of healthcare practitioners is a good first step to being able to seek the care you need and to help increase the likelihood of care coordination. So, where do you start?

Primary Care

Your primary care practitioner is typically the first point of entry into the healthcare system. Trained in general internal medicine, family medicine, or pediatrics, a primary care practitioner can provide both preventive and acute care as well as coordinate treatment when many specialists are involved.

A primary care practitioner is expected to know your medical history, to monitor your health through regular checkups over time, and to ensure you get the preventive care services you need based on your age, sex, and specific personal and family medical history. When confronted with an acute condition, your primary care practitioner can refer you to the appropriate specialist(s), if necessary, and confer with that specialist about your follow-up care. Therefore, establishing a relationship with someone who knows you and your medical history is important to do now, before you get sick.

Internal medicine (internist) vs. family medicine (family practitioner)

The main differences between an internist and a family practitioner are their medical training and therefore the type of patients they serve. Internists are trained to care for adults, whereas family practitioners gain the knowledge base to provide care to children as well. Additionally, family medicine education tends to have a greater focus on prevention and healthy lifestyles. It would also be more common to find family medicine practitioners who are comfortable performing procedures or providing such services as a pelvic exam and Pap smear or simple suturing.

You will want to select the one that feels right for you. When selecting between the two, some considerations include:

- Do you have children? If so, would you prefer an internist for you (and any other adults) and a pediatrician for your child? Or would you feel more comfortable with someone caring for the entire family?

- Do you have a complicated medical condition for which an internist might have received more comprehensive training or greater exposure during internship and residency?

Regardless of whom you choose, it is important to:

- Develop a trusting relationship and have confidence in the clinician.

- Ensure the clinician is interested in you as a whole person, not simply a collection of symptoms and diagnoses, and considers your emotional/mental health to be as important as your physical well-being.

- Make certain the clinician is open about what they do not know and are willing to seek help from other specialists when a patient's condition is beyond their expertise.

Doctor of Osteopathy (DO) vs. Doctor of Medicine (MD)[1]

A Doctor of Osteopathic Medicine (DO) is a fully licensed physician trained in a whole-person approach to medicine. A DO typically has a greater focus during training and in practice on prevention, patient education, and the impact of a patient's lifestyle and environment on well-being. DOs have additional training in the musculoskeletal system that enables them to perform some manipulations that may be similar to those one might experience when seeing a chiropractor. They have learned methods to relieve back and neck pain as well as strained muscles and are expected to participate in at least an additional two hundred hours or more of hands-on training on the musculoskeletal system ("osteopathic manipulative treatment"). Many DOs practice primary care, but they may also subspecialize in other areas, similar to MDs , depending on their particular career interests.

MDs are said to practice allopathic, or conventional, medicine, while DOs practice osteopathic medicine. MDs have a more historically traditional approach to diagnosing and treating conditions.

Both DOs and MDs have similarly rigorous educational and training requirements and must obtain state licensing to practice. They also have continuing education and certification requirements to maintain licensure.

Functional versus integrative medicine

According to the Institute for Functional Medicine, functional medicine is a model that follows "an individualized, patient-centered, science-based approach that empowers patients and practitioners to work together to address the underlying causes of disease and promote optimal wellness. It requires a detailed understanding of each patient's genetic, biochemical, and lifestyle factors and leverages that data to direct personalized treatment plans that lead to improved patient outcomes."[2]

The NIH's National Center for Complementary and Integrative Health (NCCIH) describes integrative health as bringing "conventional and complementary approaches together in a coordinated way. Integrative health also emphasizes multimodal interventions, which are two or more interventions such as conventional health care approaches (like medication, physical rehabilitation, psychotherapy), and complementary health approaches (like acupuncture, yoga, and probiotics) in various combinations, with an emphasis on treating the whole person rather than, for example, one organ system. Integrative health aims for well-coordinated care among different providers and institutions by bringing conventional and complementary approaches together to care for the whole person."[3]

Pediatrician

Pediatricians provide primary care to children, from birth up to the age of eighteen. They provide both preventive care and treatment of a broad range of childhood conditions, including physical, behavioral, and mental health issues.

Concierge physician

In a concierge practice, patients pay a monthly or annual fee to see a concierge physician. A concierge practice limits the size of its patient panel to provide easier access, more time allocated for your appointments, and more personalized care. Depending on the practice, you may receive a greater degree of involvement, the facilitation of appointments for specialty care, more comprehensive and effective coordination of care, and proactive reminders regarding preventive care.

Depending on the type of services provided, fees in 2022 ranged from $1,500 to $20,000 per year. For some practices, these fees represented the premium paid to be a patient of the practice. In others, the fee may include a bundle of services for which you would otherwise be paying out of pocket anyway if your health insurance coverage is through a high-deductible plan.

Nurse practitioner (NP)

A nurse practitioner is a registered nurse with advanced training, often a master's or doctoral degree. Nurse practitioners can provide many primary care services, including ordering diagnostic tests, writing prescriptions, and coordinating care. They can also obtain additional training that would enable them to gain expertise in a specialty area of focus.

Depending on the availability of physicians in your geographic area—for example, a rural setting—it might be easier to access a nurse practitioner than a primary care physician. And depending on the state in which you live, a nurse practitioner may be able to practice independently without a direct affiliation with a physician.

Physician assistant/associate (PA)

According to the American Academy of Physician Associates (AAPA), a physician assistant/associate is a medical professional who can diagnose illness, develop and manage treatment plans, prescribe medications, and serve as a patient's principal healthcare provider. Educated at the master's degree level, PAs receive extensive medical training with direct patient contact throughout their clinical rotations. PAs emphasize patient education, preventive care, and chronic care management and are often more accessible when you are scheduling a medical appointment.

Nurse practitioner versus physician assistant/associate

There are similarities between a physician assistant and a nurse practitioner. Both can pursue specialty areas of expertise. In certain states, both can practice independently, without a direct affiliation with or oversight by a physician, although the states where an NP can do so may not be the same ones as for a PA. Requirements for recertification and the areas of focus may also differ. For example, an NP may prefer a particular population of patients, such as pediatrics or women's health, while a PA may be certified in a specialty area like internal medicine, emergency medicine, or surgery.

Registered nurse (RN)

Registered nurses (RNs) work with doctors to provide direct care to patients. As licensed medical professionals, they are instrumental in helping to educate patients, coordinate care, and ensure that patients' needs are met. They are the ones most likely to administer immunizations and provide follow-up with the physician regarding patient phone calls. They often also serve as advocates.

Dentist (DDS or DMD)

In addition to a PCP, it's important to have a general dentist—DDS (Doctor of Dental Surgery) or DMD (Doctor of Medicine in Dentistry)—to care for and monitor your oral health. As mentioned in Chapter 2, the bacteria and inflammation from your teeth and gums can affect the health of your entire body.[4] Thus, regular visits to the dentist can provide preventive and diagnostic care to protect you from serious medical conditions or to mitigate their impact. For example, the inflammation from gum disease (periodontitis) can increase the risk of heart disease or make control of blood sugar more difficult if you have diabetes. Most dental offices include dental assistants, who help support the dentist during procedures, and dental hygienists, who can examine patients, take x-rays, perform cleanings, and provide education to patients.

For more complex procedures, a dentist may refer a patient to a specialist, with additional training beyond the four years of dental school. Dental specialists include:

- Periodontist—Treats diseases of the gums
- Endodontist—Specializes in root canals
- Prosthodontist—Restores/replaces teeth
- Orthodontist—Straightens teeth/corrects bite problems
- Oral surgeon—Performs surgery on mouth and jaw
- Pedodontist or pediatric dentist—Specializes in treating children and adolescents

Medical Specialists

There are many conditions that require additional training and specialization, and your primary care practitioner should be able to refer you to the appropriate specialist if your condition requires specific expertise, skill, and experience. Depending on the condition's severity, the specialist may continue to manage your treatment and should communicate with your primary care physician about your care.

There are many specialties—and subspecialties—in medicine and surgery. Here's a list of some medical specialties, along with a sample of the conditions they treat. It is impossible to include a comprehensive list of conditions, so consult your primary care practitioner for your specific situation.

Specialist	Area(s) of Focus	Some Examples of When You Might Need One
Allergist/ Immunologist	Treatment of asthma, allergies & some diseases of the immune system	An allergic reaction, such as a rash, perhaps triggered by pollen, animal dander, insect stings, latex, or mold
		Food or seasonal allergies
		Hay fever
		Eczema
		Autoimmune disorders
		Immunodeficiency conditions

Specialist	Area(s) of Focus	Some Examples of When You Might Need One
Behavioral Health Practitioners Psychologist Therapist or Counselor Clinical social worker Mental health nurse practitioner Psychiatrist	Mental & emotional health conditions The type of practitioner may vary depending on training, licensure & state of practice, the scope of conditions addressed & the ability to write prescriptions & manage medications	Depression Anxiety Stress PTSD (post-traumatic stress disorder) Bipolar disorder Schizophrenia
Cardiologist	Heart disease, heart abnormalities & other diseases of the cardiovascular system	Tightness or pain in your chest, arm, neck, or back Lightheadedness, shortness of breath, nausea, or heart palpitations A cardiologist may refer you to a cardiac surgeon for complex procedures.
Dermatologist	Skin disorders—including hair & nails—such as eczema & psoriasis	A full-body skin check is advised to catch potential melanoma, or skin cancer, in its early stages. A small piece of skin may be removed to biopsy if a skin area looks suspicious.
Endocrinologist	Disorders of the endocrine glands & hormones	Types 1 & 2 diabetes Thyroid disease Infertility Growth issues
Gastroenterologist/ GI	Problems of the entire digestive system including the stomach, intestines, liver, gallbladder & pancreas	Diverticulitis Inflammatory bowel disease Irritable bowel syndrome May perform colonoscopies to screen for colon cancer A gastroenterologist may refer you to a colorectal surgeon to perform more specialized surgery of the rectum, anus & intestinal tract.
Gerontologist/ geriatrician	Issues related to aging & the biological, cognitive, psychological & sociological concerns of the elderly	Alzheimer's Parkinson's Depression Anxiety End-of-life issues

Specialist	Area(s) of Focus	Some Examples of When You Might Need One
Gynecologist	Female reproductive system	Pelvic exams Cancer screening Endometriosis Ovarian cysts Fibroids Vaginal infections & concerns related to sexual health Hysterectomy
Hematologist	Disorders related to blood, bone marrow & the lymphatic system	Cancers of the blood such as leukemia or multiple myeloma Anemia (low red blood cells) Deep vein thrombosis (blood clots)
Hepatologist	Specializes in diseases of the liver & bile ducts	Hepatitis Wilson's disease
Hospitalist	Specializes in the medical care of hospitalized patients	Direct patient care Care coordination & communication during a hospital stay
Infectious disease specialist	Diseases caused by microorganisms, such as bacteria & viruses	HIV/AIDS Tuberculosis Pneumonia Tropical diseases, such as malaria The coronavirus
Nephrologist	Diseases of the kidney	Kidney infections & kidney failure
Neurologist	Disorders of the brain, spinal cord & peripheral nerves & muscles	Migraines Epilepsy Stroke Multiple sclerosis (MS) Parkinson's Consult a neurologist if you are having persistent head pain, memory loss, tremors, or lack of balance & coordination. You may be referred to a neurosurgeon to perform surgery on the brain, spinal cord, or the central nervous system.

Specialist	Area(s) of Focus	Some Examples of When You Might Need One
Obstetrician	Pregnancy Childbirth & postpartum care Often combined with gynecology	If you suspect you are pregnant or are within the first six to eight weeks, to ensure proper prenatal care
Oncologist	Diagnosis & treatment of cancer	May treat cancer through medication, chemotherapy, radiation & other targeted therapies such as immunotherapy
Ophthalmologist	Disorders & diseases of the eye	If you are experiencing a loss of vision, flashes of light, double vision, streaks, distortions, pain, swelling, or changes in the field of vision, see an ophthalmologist. Conditions include glaucoma, cataracts, age-related macular degeneration & diabetic eye disease. They are different from optometrists, who can provide primary care for the eye, identify a vision problem & prescribe glasses or corrective lenses. Opticians fill prescriptions & ensure that eyeglasses or contact lenses fit correctly.
Orthopedist/ orthopedic surgeon	The skeletal & muscular system including bones, joints, muscles, cartilage, ligaments & tendons	Hip or knee replacement Herniated disc Injury with broken bones
Otolaryngologist/ ear, nose & throat (ENT)	Diseases of the ears, nose, throat, head & neck	Chronic ear or sinus infection Deviated septum Bronchitis Tonsil removal Vocal cord disorders

Specialist	Area(s) of Focus	Some Examples of When You Might Need One
Plastic surgeon	Repair or reconstruction of physical defects, particularly those involving the skin, face, hand, breast & musculoskeletal system	Reduce scarring or disfigurement resulting from accidents, birth defects, or melanomas Also perform elective cosmetic surgery Reconstructive surgeons may take tissue from one area of your body to repair another area, for example, taking bone from your leg to repair a jaw.
Podiatrist	Treatment of the foot, ankles & lower legs	Fungal toenail infections Corns Calluses Bunions Athlete's foot Foot problems due to diabetes
Pulmonologist	Diseases of the respiratory system & lung disorders	Chronic breathing problems Respiratory infections COPD (chronic obstructive pulmonary disease)
Radiologist	Uses medical imaging, such as x-rays, CT scans (computerized tomography) & MRIs (magnetic resonance imaging), to diagnose disease	Mammogram to detect breast cancer Ultrasound to check the health of a fetus Echocardiogram to evaluate your heart functioning
Rheumatologist	Treats arthritis, along with other musculoskeletal conditions & autoimmune diseases, when the immune system produces unnecessary inflammation in the body	Rheumatoid & psoriatic arthritis Lupus Osteoarthritis & gout Often, these conditions persist for a long time, so it's important to seek treatment promptly.
Surgeon	Uses surgical procedures to diagnose & remove disease, repair injuries & promote healing. May specialize in certain parts of the body, for example, colorectal, thoracic, orthopedic	Cancer Gallstones Appendicitis Hernia Varicose veins Non-cancerous tumors, nodules, or cysts Rectal incontinence

Specialist	Area(s) of Focus	Some Examples of When You Might Need One
Urogynecologist	Treats problems that affect female pelvic floor conditions	Weak or overactive bladder Pelvic organ prolapse (weak pelvic muscles) Bladder incontinence
Urologist	Disorders of the urinary system, particularly those involving the kidneys, bladder & prostate	Urinary tract infections (UTIs) Kidney stones A urologist also specializes in the male reproductive system & may perform an exam to evaluate the prostate.

Finding the Right Specialist

Finding the right specialist can be difficult, especially if you are in a geographical area with limited options. Your primary care practitioner should help identify and refer you to the appropriate specialist for your specialty care needs.

If you have arrived in the emergency room with an acute medical condition or are admitted to the hospital, a specialist may be consulted to determine next steps, whether you need to be admitted or observed, and, depending on the condition, to be primarily responsible for managing your care.

But if you do have a choice, how do you find the right one for you? As will be discussed in Chapter 4, partnering with your healthcare practitioner is critical to your health and well-being. It may take a few visits to establish this relationship and to know you are in the right hands.

- Seeking a referral from your primary care physician is a good place to start. As mentioned before, this may also help to ensure better overall coordination of your care when several clinicians are involved.

- Reach out to other healthcare professionals to obtain their recommendations. They may have experience working with specific providers and have observed firsthand how the specialists care for their patients. While recommendations from friends and family can be helpful, be cautious, as their experiences may not be the same as yours.

- Ratings from local publications or certain websites like Healthgrades.com may be somewhat helpful, but reflect the various perceptions and differing experiences patients can have. They may not contain objective data about the number of procedures performed, successful outcomes, and other pertinent information about the physician's performance.

- Look for a hospital that specializes in your condition. Their physicians may be leading the latest research and may be more aware of the most current treatment options.

- Check with your state licensing board. It may be able to provide information like formal complaints, malpractice lawsuit history, or history of licensure suspension.

No matter whom you choose, communication among healthcare practitioners is important. Those who work as a team are usually your best option. Ask about how they confer and work together to determine the most appropriate treatment plan for you. Find out how they will partner with you in the decision-making process.

Selecting the Right Provider for You

Selecting healthcare practitioners is a personal experience. It is important, if you have a variety of options, that you choose individuals who not only are well trained and experienced but also are a good fit for you. As you meet with different healthcare practitioners, consider asking some of the following questions to find the right one(s) for you (see Chapter 4 for more on this issue):

- What is the provider's philosophy of care, and do you share that philosophy? For example, are you looking for a more holistic and preventive approach to your health and well-being, or a more targeted one focused mainly on treating your chronic or acute conditions? Is the provider willing to work with your health beliefs, even in instances when they may differ from their own?

- How accessible is the provider? Are you able to reach them via email or text with a question in addition to contacting the office? And are there safety precautions—for example, encrypted systems—in place to ensure protection of your data and during exchanges of the digital variety?

- How are emergencies handled? Can you be seen quickly if there's an acute condition? What call coverage system is in place when the practitioner is not available?

- What hospitals are the providers affiliated with? Are those hospitals accessible and highly rated for your condition?

- Depending on your insurance plan, is the provider in the network? Are you willing to pay more to see those who are out-of-network? Be sure the provider accepts your insurance (e.g., some do not accept Medicare or all insurance company health plans), and if not, decide if you are willing to pay more (or completely out-of-pocket if they do not take insurance at all) to see those who are out-of-network.

- Is there an electronic health record (EHR) or electronic medical record (EMR) system for documenting your personal medical information including visits, test results, medications, allergies, etc., and how easy and secure is it to access? Is there a tracking system to make you aware of any preventive care, such as immunizations and cancer screenings? Is this EHR/EMR used by most of your physicians? Can you easily use the EHR/EMR to ask your provider a question through a patient portal?

- Are there virtual care/telehealth capabilities for appointments that do not require an in-person visit?

- Will prescription refills and special requests (e.g., proof of immunization for school or camp) be handled promptly?

Often, your decision may be a subjective one and greatly influenced by the quality of the interaction between you and the provider.

Some Things to Consider When Making a Decision

- Do you feel respected, or was the interaction condescending or patronizing?

- Do you feel comfortable asking questions?
- Were you made aware of all your options? Does the provider seem open to other treatment options, such as acupuncture?
- Were you involved in the decision-making about your treatment plan?
- Is the provider a good listener and interested in learning more about you?
- Did the provider seem interested in your emotional/mental health (e.g., stress or anxiety), or did the conversation just focus on physical issues?
- Did the conversation focus on your areas of concern and not just the ones the provider wanted to cover? Were all your concerns addressed?
- Were the explanations clear? Did the provider minimize the medical jargon and ensure you understood? Were the instructions about medications and the treatment plan made very clear?

Bottom line, you want to select a healthcare practitioner with whom you feel comfortable and who you can trust to deliver the best possible care. To develop that trust, you must be actively involved in your care, share complete information, and participate in the decision-making process. When all is said and done, you are in charge of your own health and well-being!

SO, WHAT CAN YOU DO NOW?

- The complexity of health and the healthcare system can be intimidating and challenging to decipher. Your PCP is a good starting point to help you navigate.

- Regardless of the type of healthcare professional, good communication, trust, and respect are critical. Select a primary care practitioner who is experienced and a good fit for you.

- If your care involves several healthcare practitioners, make sure you know who is leading the team and coordinating your care.

- If you have symptoms that are not getting better or are becoming worse, if the diagnosis is a dilemma, or if your gut is telling you to pursue things further, you may need the additional expertise of a specialist or a second opinion. Your PCP should be able to provide a referral to a specialist.

CHAPTER 4

Partnering with Your Doctor

In my view, the lost art of listening, and ignoring the patient as a human being is a quintessential failure of our health care.

BERNARD LOWN, MD

CHARLENE'S STORY, CONTINUED

Four years after my fifth surgery related to the brain tumor and many months of antibiotics, I experienced another health concern in April 2014. I became extremely fatigued, with a dry, unproductive cough that wouldn't go away.

After two weeks of continued symptoms, I decided it was time to call my primary care physician (PCP), who promptly referred me to an ear, nose, and throat (ENT) specialist. The specialist couldn't find anything wrong. I returned to my PCP, who then ordered a blood test. The test revealed that my C-reactive protein (CRP) and sed rate (erythrocyte sedimentation rate, or ESR) levels were highly elevated, both indications of inflammation. But where in my body was the inflammation?

Over the following ten days, I was referred to several different specialists to find the problem. It became clear to me that medicine has become extremely specialized when a cardiologist declared, "Your heart is fine; that's all I can tell you." He couldn't speculate about what else could be causing the problem.

My last visit was to an oncologist, who also found nothing wrong but suggested I get a chest x-ray. The x-ray revealed that my arteries—blood vessels that carry oxygen-rich blood away from the heart to the body—were inflamed.

My PCP referred me to a rheumatologist, who made a diagnosis of an autoimmune disorder called "giant cell arteritis." Typically, the symptoms include headaches, jaw pain, and fever, none of which I had experienced. The treatment for this condition is steroid medication, and I was put on a daily 60 milligram dose of prednisone. The cough disappeared immediately, but the prednisone made me edgy, as if I were jumping out of my skin. It interfered with my sleep, and I began to gain weight. While the physician was very polite and responsive, he thought it would be best if I saw the chief rheumatologist at the nearby large teaching hospital in the city, the "expert" in his field.

The chief rheumatologist's manner was efficient and to the point. He asked very few questions about me personally or about my medical history, nor did he seem to invite any questions.

He added another medication, methotrexate, to my regimen. I told him, given my previous history with so many antibiotics and the side effects of the prednisone, I was reluctant to take yet another pill. He promptly dismissed my concern. "Methotrexate has been used safely for years," he assured me. "This is standard protocol. However, because these medications suppress your immune system, you should refrain from plane travel and be sure to get a flu shot." *Good advice*, I thought, and so I complied; yet I continued to experience the negative side effects.

After several months on the prednisone and methotrexate, I gained an additional fifteen pounds, and my face grew puffy. I continued to get blood tests to monitor my CRP and sed rate, and eventually the levels began to diminish. The doctor began to slowly decrease the amount of medication.

At about the one-year point, a routine blood test indicated both my CRP and sed rate had increased slightly, and the chief rheumatologist wanted me to return to the previous high dosage of prednisone. I had been feeling much better overall and was reluctant to go through the debilitating side effects of the steroid all over again. I was at a crossroads and unsure what to do.

"I'd like to get a second opinion," I stated.

"There can only be one captain of this ship!" he snapped back. "But, if you insist, I will give you the name of another physician."

I was stunned by his reaction. Was I making a mistake about my own health? Wasn't he the expert in the field?

I decided not to call the physician he suggested. Frankly, I had a low expectation that he would disagree. I thought perhaps some physicians would be reluctant to render a different opinion and would defer to the "expert."

Instead, I contacted another physician whom I had seen in the past. After reviewing my medical records, he encouraged me to move forward with a second opinion. Through a contact in the patient relations department of a hospital in another city one hour away, I was given the name of an experienced, highly regarded rheumatologist.

I had seen many wonderful physicians throughout my life for whom I had developed deep respect and admiration, and I immediately felt I was in the right hands with this physician. This initial visit had a profound impact on me—not because of the ease of access, the efficiency of the office, or any modern technology, but because of the humility, the sincerity, and the communication style of the physician.

First, he took the time to ask many questions and truly listened. He wanted to know what I was experiencing, how I felt, and what, if anything, had changed. He reviewed my family medical history in detail, even though it was captured on paper. At the end of the conversation, he probed further, "What else about your medical history might be relevant that we haven't talked about so far?"

He wanted to get to know me as a person. He prodded. "Tell me about you." I glanced at my husband, who had accompanied me, for an answer. "She likes to make things happen," my husband joked, "and she likes to be the boss." We all had a good laugh.

The physician wanted to know about my profession, what I liked to do for recreation, and what was important to me. He took a holistic view of my health and asked, "What is your diet like?" and "Tell me about your exercise routine."

He shared his own personal philosophy. He explained that his father was a country physician and said he learned to listen and communicate by accompanying his father on house calls. He shared the following quote of Sir William Osler, often called the Father of Modern Medicine: "The good physician treats the disease; the great physician treats the patient who has the disease."

My physical examination was also quite different. He examined me to look for other physical indicators that would suggest a return of the disease, such as taking my blood pressure in both arms and comparing the two. He explained what he was looking for, and his explanations were clear and easily understandable without talking down to me. He said we were partners in my care and that I was the senior partner.

Toward the end of the visit, he asked, "What else do I need to know about you in order to provide the best possible care?" I didn't know what else to say other than "thank you." He gave me his cell phone number in case I needed to contact him urgently, something most doctors would not typically do out of concern that it could be misused. He ordered some additional blood tests and said he would call me the next day as soon as the results were in—and he did.

As a result of that visit and the review of my tests, he said he did not believe the inflammation had returned. While he complimented my previous physician for getting me to this point, he recommended I reduce the amount of medication, not increase it. My instincts were confirmed, and I was totally relieved.

Did I continue to see this physician because he told me what I wanted to hear? Not really. It was more because he took the time to understand me, and he had an easy, empathetic communication style. His patient-centered approach felt like a true partnership, unlike that of the former chief rheumatologist who conveyed a message that said, "I'm the expert; just do as I say." I asked the nurse if he treats all his patients this way, particularly the ones who are less fortunate. She confirmed that he did.

Fortunately, my symptoms resolved after being slowly weaned from the medication. I continue to see this physician periodically to ensure the autoimmune disorder remains in remission. I feel very blessed to have such a special physician who truly knows how to put Osler's words into practice.

LESSONS LEARNED

- Charlene was fortunate to find a physician with whom she could partner. Finding the physician who is right for you may require some trial and error. Look for a physician who listens, asks questions, and cares about you as a person, not just a condition.

- Getting to the correct diagnosis is not always easy and may take persistence. Be willing to ask for a second opinion.

- Don't be afraid to question the proposed treatment if you don't feel comfortable or are not sure it's the right one for you.

- Trust and respect are key to a successful partnership with your physician.

WHAT YOU NEED TO KNOW

Most physicians are well-meaning and truly care about the well-being of their patients. However, the physician-patient experience is often far from being a partnership. True partnerships, both personal and professional, are characterized by mutual trust and respect, open and honest two-way communication, a shared commitment to common goals, and joint decision-making.

Some physicians hurry through appointments due to heavy workloads and fail to engage their patients in meaningful conversations about their care. Some physicians don't take the time to truly listen, and their demeanor can make it difficult to ask questions.

Of course, physicians are human and sometimes may forget or neglect to follow up. From the physician's perspective, they may be trying to deal with office management issues, such as staffing shortages, high turnover, and reimbursement challenges. There could be a lack of technical expertise and perhaps an insufficient infrastructure around reminder systems for preventive care or HIPAA-compliant platforms for telehealth and email communication. And certainly COVID-19 has made things that much more difficult for healthcare professionals in general.

Although there has been some improvement, medical and other health professional schools often have limited training on critical communication skills, such as how to draw out a patient's priorities and values and to listen nonjudgmentally to support positive changes in the patient's life. Training for healthcare professionals often has not focused on building such skills as expressing empathy, showing humility, and displaying cultural sensitivity.

Health disparities and power dynamics in a clinical setting have typically been given minimal attention. Moreover, as the recent pandemic has shown, clinicians have experienced a major increase in burnout themselves and often have not received sufficient support to help maintain their own health and well-being.

Patients can often feel intimidated. Just entering a medical environment can cause stress and anxiety, such as, "white coat syndrome," the sudden spike in blood pressure some people experience when they visit a doctor. Even the most well-educated and savvy individuals can feel out of their element when face-to-face with a physician. And there is a phenomenon (often generational) in which some patients believe the doctor knows best; therefore, it would be inappropriate to question or challenge their opinion. As evident in the patient story, it was difficult to question the physician's proposed treatment.

Additionally, patients often lack self-advocacy skills and may possess limited health literacy (which is *not* the same as general literacy). They may have insufficient knowledge of their bodies to be comfortable about taking charge of their health and well-being. Lacking the resources to navigate a complex and often unfriendly healthcare system, their healthcare interactions are often fraught with emotions of fear and feelings of helplessness.

With all the wonderful advances in medical research and technological innovations, we know the communication between the physician and the patient is critical to a correct diagnosis and a positive health outcome. As Sir William Osler wisely said, "Listen to your patient, he is telling you the diagnosis." Better communication can lead to a greater ability to diagnose a health problem, to do so more quickly, to increase the understanding of treatment options, and to increase adherence to the treatment plan itself.

If you have questions or concerns after leaving the physician's office, you can usually communicate with your physician through a phone call to the office or an email to the practice. It is important to be clear about the reason for your call and how time-sensitive the issue is. Many practices may take several days to return your call. In the case of an urgent situation after normal business hours, you would most often be directed to contact an answering service who will reach out to the clinician on call. In the case of an emergency, you will typically be directed to go to the emergency room.

Communicating through a Patient Portal

Many healthcare providers, group medical practices, and hospital systems use an online website to store medical records and to communicate with patients. Accessed with a secure username and password, patients can use the portal to confirm appointments, send and receive messages, view recent visit summaries, and update information about medications, immunizations, and allergies. Patients have the right to obtain their data from healthcare providers as quickly as possible, which is often accomplished via a patient portal.

While patient portals can be beneficial, they are not designed for situations in which a medical condition is urgent, or you need to communicate with a physician immediately. Depending on how often providers check their messages, response times may vary. It's a good idea to ask if the provider uses the patient portal regularly and considers it an important resource. If your healthcare provider has incorporated it into the daily workflow, you may be able to save time and get a more rapid response.

The portals are also used to get results from lab tests, x-rays, pathology reports, and other important assessments. These test results may be loaded into the portal and sometimes appear before the doctor has an opportunity to review and discuss them with the patient. Because medical information can be complicated and difficult to understand, a patient may have questions and perhaps misinterpret the results. For example, a patient may think a lab result indicates cancer and could become very distressed, even though cancer might not be present at all.

While some patients appreciate knowing the results of tests as soon as they are available, others may find it confusing. Therefore, it is important to determine whether you want to view the results in the portal immediately, or to wait until you can discuss them with your provider.

Beginning the Partnership

First, be open and share your complete medical history, all symptoms, and any medications. Recently, I learned of a patient who was reluctant to tell her doctor she was seeing a psychiatrist and taking an antidepressant because of the stigma attached to mental illness. Withholding information, even if you think it's unrelated, can affect the type of treatment selected and result in adverse effects from medication combinations that can be deadly.

Talk about your goals and expectations. Share what you hope to achieve—for example, to play the piano again, to play golf, to walk down the aisle at your daughter's wedding. In severe cases, where full recovery may not be possible, sometimes a physician can help you achieve a more modest goal.

Ask questions to get the information you need to feel comfortable with your care. For example:

- "Help me understand the severity of my condition, my treatment options, and the likely outcomes of each." If you don't understand any medical jargon, don't hesitate to ask for a clearer explanation. Ask for any literature you can read later that might provide additional information and reinforce instructions you may have been given.

- "How do I get in touch with you if I have an important question or problem? If I reach voicemail or an answering service, how soon can I expect a reply? If you're unavailable, whom do I contact?"

- "How much will this procedure cost? Are there less expensive treatment options that work as well?" You may be directed to the office manager or billing personnel to get information regarding the cost of services.

- If there are other physicians involved, "Who will coordinate my care? How will you be following up with them and communicating with each other?"

- "Are there community resources or social worker services available to help provide support?"

Knowing that physicians are not infallible and cannot provide 100 percent guarantees, it's important to ask for and discuss all treatment options and the anticipated pros and cons of each. As a patient, you must fully understand your role in adhering to the treatment plan and follow up. If you think you cannot follow through with the proposed plan, or it is not one that is a fit for you, speak up, and jointly agree on a path forward that is doable given your circumstances and health beliefs.

Disclose any personal situations at home or at work that might be impacting your health. For example:

- Do you live alone and need help during recovery after an operation?

- Are you worried about caring for children, elderly parents, or pets when you're sick?
- Are you experiencing undue stress at work, or afraid you will lose employment while in the hospital or recovering at home?
- Are you worried about the financial burden? How will the out-of-pocket costs influence your treatment decisions?

Even if you think the information is not relevant, share these concerns with your doctor. You may be missing out on services that can help during your treatment and recovery.

THINGS TO DISCUSS WITH YOUR DOCTOR

- If you are concerned about anything, just ask. Don't be afraid to disclose something that you think may be embarrassing. The doctor has probably heard and seen it before.

- Pay attention to your body. You know it best. Even if it seems minor, let the doctor know about any unusual signs or symptoms that could be an indication of a new or serious medical condition.

- State what medications or supplements you are taking and why you are taking them. Tell the doctor about the dosage, and when and how you're taking them (e.g., time of day, with meals, etc.). How are they working? Any side effects?

- Communicate your family medical history. What medical conditions did your parents and immediate family members have? If deceased, what were the causes of their deaths?

- Share your own medical history, including any past health issues that could be impacting you today.

- Lifestyle is important. Talk about your eating habits, whether you smoke now or have in the past, the number of alcoholic beverages you typically drink, how much regular physical activity you get, your normal sleep patterns, and your level of stress. These can all impact the diagnosis and treatment plan for your medical condition.

- Remember that everyone is different and unique. You can discuss a friend or relative's treatment but understand it may not work the same for you. Figure out the appropriate treatment plan together with your doctor.

- Feel free to ask about a drug advertisement on TV or a health article on the internet but realize that it may not be totally accurate. It's best if you can talk through the research and make an informed decision together.

- Show your understanding that a doctor's day can go awry, too. If the doctor has a more urgent situation and must reschedule an appointment, work together to find a convenient time. If the doctor forgets to share information or didn't get a chance to follow up with you, don't hesitate to speak up.

- Finally, share anything else you think the doctor needs to know about you to give you the best possible care.

Creating a partnership with your doctor requires good interpersonal skills on the part of both individuals. Often called social skills, people skills, or "soft" skills, they are well developed by the most effective physicians, who know the importance of interacting to build trust and assure patients they are in good hands. We often refer to this as "bedside manner," which patients judge as a major indicator of their doctors' general competence.[1] It includes not only good communication skills but also "emotional intelligence." For example, how does the physician manage their own emotions and sense the emotions of others? How does the physician show empathy and handle a patient who is anxious or upset?

As patients, we need to understand that doctors are human, too. They have good days and bad days, and their personal lives can intrude into their workday just like they sometimes do for all of us. When emergencies arise, they run late through no fault of their own. Explaining these possibilities upfront makes it easier for patients to be understanding, extend grace, and remain flexible when schedules get adjusted and unavoidable delays occur.

Some physicians experience stress and burnout in their jobs because of the constant demands on their time, juggling multiple patients and responsibilities, and the frustration of sometimes not being able to heal or save a life. We have become painfully aware of how healthcare workers on the frontlines of the pandemic have coped with the grueling nature of their jobs. As patients, we must show patience and empathy as well. Just as we want doctors to be sensitive to our needs, we also need to recognize theirs.

However, when a physician is consistently rushed, disinterested, dismissive, or even rude, a change is warranted if you have that option. A patient relayed the following experience: "In one initial office visit, the doctor was scrolling through his emails on his phone—with no explanation—while I was conveying my medical history. I don't know if he was looking for an urgent message or not, but I left the office gracefully and never returned."

Asking for a Second Opinion

You may have a deep trust in a physician's competence but not be comfortable with the recommended treatment plan. And, as described in the patient story, some physicians may not make it easy to question what they consider their authority. In such a situation, it may take courage to obtain a second opinion, although this can be easier said than done. Here are some reasons why patients are hesitant to ask for a second opinion:

- *"I don't want the doctor to think I don't trust them. I don't want the doctor to think I'm challenging their judgment."* Patients trust their healthcare providers and can be reluctant to question their treatment recommendations. Asking for a second opinion might be interpreted as a loss of confidence in the physician's abilities.

- *"I don't want to be perceived as a difficult patient or appear rude."* Patients want the doctor to feel good about them and don't want to potentially damage the relationship. For example, if they are about to undergo surgery, patients want to make sure the doctor likes them and will take special care of them throughout the entire process.

- *"My doctor's office is so busy. There are so many patients waiting to see them, and there is so little time for me as it is.*

If I ask to have all my records sent, it's just creating extra work for the entire staff." Again, some patients don't want to seem difficult and are reluctant to ask for anything that might be perceived as an unnecessary inconvenience to the physician or the staff.

- *"English is not my native language, and I don't completely understand what he's saying. I probably should see a physician who can explain things to me in my own language."* Patients may withhold personal information out of a feeling of confusion or embarrassment or may misinterpret the questions that are being asked.

- *"My doctor is recommending a particular procedure that will cost me a lot of money. I'm not sure whether I should put the treatment off and first research what the typical price for this procedure is. I am reluctant to say this to the doctor."* Patients may not want to question a doctor's fees but may feel that the cost is too high. As a result, some may want to postpone the procedure or see if there are other options. They may wonder if there are significant differences in what providers charge.

- *"The doctor is just going to give me the name of a friend or colleague. The second physician won't want to throw my doctor under the bus."* Patients may not know whom to contact and may believe a second physician will not contradict a colleague out of respect, professional courtesy, referral patterns, or office politics.

- *"I know there is no hope for a different outcome, so it would be a waste of time. Besides, I don't have the time to travel far to get another opinion."* After a serious diagnosis, some patients are understandably sad and despondent. They may feel a sense of futility in seeking another solution to their health problem. They may also feel pressured by a sense of urgency to begin treatment and choose to forgo the exploration of other potential options.

You have the right to ask for another perspective about your medical care. As in the previous patient story, pursuing a second opinion can help ensure that you better understand your options and feel more secure about moving forward, and hopefully can lead to an optimal outcome.

Dealing with Possible Mistakes

Medicine is an art as well as a science. The same medication, procedure, or treatment can have very different results among people with the same condition. A healthcare practitioner can do everything by the book, and still an unsuccessful outcome can result. However, well-trained physicians and other healthcare providers are not infallible, and mistakes do occur. For example, according to a May 2022 report by the Office of Inspector General (OIG) of the Department of Health and Human Services, 25 percent of Medicare patients hospitalized in October 2018 experienced adverse and temporary harm events.[2]

This does not necessarily mean healthcare practitioners are bad or incompetent. Rather, the researchers say errors are more likely due to a lack of coordination in the healthcare system and the "absence or underuse" of standard safety protocols and practices. Sometimes there's an incomplete handoff from one practitioner to another without ample communication or information, or there could be a lack of communication across the entire healthcare team regarding a patient's treatment. This seemed to be the case in Charlene's story in the introduction.

Maximizing your safety

- Don't assume all healthcare practitioners involved in your care have communicated with each other. Confirm that medical records have been shared and received. Ensure that your primary care practitioner follows up with any specialists and is informed of any medication changes, procedures, or follow-up treatment.

THE OFFICE OF INSPECTOR GENERAL (OIG) DEFINES CERTAIN TYPES OF MISTAKES THAT CAN OCCUR DURING HOSPITALIZATION.[3]

- Adverse event—An event, preventable or nonpreventable, that caused harm to a patient due to medical care. This includes hospital-acquired conditions, events that required life-sustaining intervention, and events that caused prolonged hospital stays, permanent harm, or death.

- Never event—A serious event, such as surgery on the wrong patient, that the National Quality Forum included on a specific list of events that "should never occur in a health care setting."

- Temporary harm event—An event that requires intervention but does not cause lasting harm; examples are an allergic reaction or hypoglycemia.

- Ensure that you are fully informed about exactly what is about to happen, and check your understanding. Before any surgical procedures, ask the surgeon to confirm what is being removed, repaired, or replaced. Take any forms seriously, and read them in detail before signing.

- If you receive conflicting or confusing information, ask questions for clarification, and express your concerns. If the provider seems rushed or distracted, ask them to slow down, and, if necessary, schedule another appointment to complete the conversation.

- Before you get an injection or take medication, confirm what you're getting, and why. Ask about any possible adverse reactions and what to do in the event they occur. Be sure you know how to take your medications and ask if there are any foods or drinks you should avoid when taking them. Also, ask about any potential drug interactions. Your pharmacist may also be able to provide some valuable information.

- If you don't feel comfortable with the person treating you, or if you think the person is doing something wrong or needs help (for example, the person is having difficulty inserting an IV), you may need to ask for another provider.

- Don't be afraid to ask for a second opinion.

- Take notes during appointments, and ask questions to confirm your understanding.

- If you are hospitalized and concerned about your care, ask to see a patient advocate. They should be able to help address your needs.

Lastly, it is important to understand that poor outcomes or complications do not necessarily mean there were any errors in the care delivered. For example, surgery does carry some potential risk. That's why it is important to make sure you understand all the possible risks and benefits of your care and make an informed decision that is best for your situation.

A true patient-physician partnership—one in which you both communicate freely and make decisions jointly—can result in a more satisfying and less stressful experience for both the patient and the physician. Trust and less stress can also lead to better health outcomes and lower out-of-pocket costs for the patient, including better management of chronic conditions, more care focused on prevention, fewer ER visits, shorter hospital stays, improved treatment plan adherence, and a speedier recovery. More satisfied patients can contribute to less burnout and greater job satisfaction for physicians as well.

Under ideal circumstances, you will have a relationship with your healthcare providers marked by compassion, mutual trust, honesty, and respect. It is important to recognize your role and responsibility to help your caregivers provide the best possible care.

SO, WHAT CAN YOU DO NOW?

- Make a list of questions to ask your physician at your next visit. If you are worried about a particular issue, don't hesitate to raise the concern.

- Be willing to share your health beliefs, concerns, and any obstacles that may make it challenging to follow the medical advice you are given.

- If you believe that your physician is not listening or is ignoring your concerns, be prepared to speak up or bring a family member or friend who can speak on your behalf. If you are feeling intimidated and not comfortable with the physician, research other available practitioners.

- Look for a practitioner who can provide a second opinion.

- Make sure the doctor providing the second opinion has your full medical records including any x-rays, test results, and other relevant information.

- Speak up if you suspect a mistake has been made. Be vigilant in all healthcare settings to reduce the risk of a medical error.

CHAPTER 5

Coordinating Care

Providing healthcare is like building a house. The task requires experts, expensive equipment and materials, and a huge amount of coordination.

ATUL GAWANDE, MD

ANN'S STORY

Ann and her husband, Don, were university professors in Hawaii teaching classes in special education. As parents of a son with cerebral palsy, they knew firsthand the challenges of raising a child with special needs. With four additional children, Ann had learned the importance of staying positive and resilient for the entire family. However, that resilience was put to the test when she faced her own health issues.

At age sixty-two, Ann agreed in 2005 to teach a class on the island of Tutuila in Samoa. While in Samoa, she made many friends and enjoyed sewing as a pastime. During one stay in Samoa, Ann noticed that her legs were different sizes. Using the tape measure from her sewing kit, Ann discovered that her left thigh, knee, and ankle were one inch bigger than the right.

Medical services were meager on the island, and by the time she returned to Hawaii, her left leg had grown four inches larger than the right. Her general practitioner thought she might have caught some tropical disease. He ordered a sonogram, but it revealed nothing.

Back home, Ann suddenly developed severe back pain and had difficulty urinating. Don rushed her to the emergency room. The doctors thought she had developed a blood clot. They immediately gave her Lovenox, a blood thinner, and surgically implanted an aortic filter to keep the blood clot from traveling to her heart.

Discharged from the hospital, Ann noticed that her stomach was getting bruised and growing larger. Her trouble urinating continued. Still in pain, Ann and her husband decided to go back to the emergency room. At the hospital, a stent was placed in her ureter, and they took a biopsy of her groin.

After admission to the hospital, Ann was seen by many healthcare professionals—an oncologist, a radiologist, a nephrologist, a urologist, a gastroenterologist, an endocrinologist, and a hospitalist—to figure out what was going on. She was eventually diagnosed with non-Hodgkin's lymphoma, a type of cancer that starts in the white blood cells and affects the body's lymph and immune systems.

During her three weeks in the hospital, Don kept a journal of everything related to Ann's case, because she was in no condition to remember the many conversations with all the physicians. Don's meticulous notes helped clarify instructions and allowed them to question any comments that seemed contradictory.

One event that Don recorded in his journal was the "Dance of the Nurses," as he called it. Ann was scheduled for a chemotherapy infusion; however, it wasn't clear which nurse was supposed to administer the treatment. The hospital's infusion center was an outpatient arm of the hospital, and since Ann was an inpatient, the nurse from the infusion center wanted the nurse on the floor to administer the chemo. Apparently neither wanted to do it, and they started to argue about whose responsibility it was, in front of Ann and her husband. Their bickering was disturbing to say the least, and Don finally called the director of nursing to resolve the dispute.

About a week later, Ann's sister Kay flew in from the East Coast and arrived at the hospital by 9:30 p.m., just in time to witness one of the hospitalists rudely speaking to Ann at her bedside. The hospitalist barked, "What are you still doing in the hospital? We have sicker patients than you that need this room. I am discharging you right away. You'll have to give yourself the Lovenox shots at home."

"I don't know if I can do that myself," Ann cried. Meanwhile, Don wondered, "I don't even know if the pharmacy is open at this hour to get the medication."

Confused and upset, her husband and sister took Ann home. But at 3:00 a.m., they brought her back to the hospital because Ann was still in severe pain, and she discovered blood in her urine. Ann remained in the ICU for several days. Before she was moved to the step-down unit, Don and Kay insisted that the hospitalist who had discharged her previously be excluded from her case. The hospital agreed.

With so many different physicians treating her, Ann was perplexed about who was ultimately responsible for her care. Don arranged for her primary care physician (PCP), who drove thirty miles to the hospital, to become her "case manager." Her PCP spoke to each of the specialists and coordinated her treatment. When one of the doctors wanted to insert a port to administer medicine, Ann asked if her PCP had been consulted. "Yes, he approved it," she was told.

Now confident that someone whom she trusted was managing her care, Ann's anxiety began to subside. However, Ann was still worried about the bruising and swelling of her stomach. As a result of the Lovenox injections, a hematoma about the size of a human head and containing 1800 cubic centimeters of blood had collected in her gut.

"Why are you still giving the blood thinner to her?" Don asked. "She doesn't have a blood clot, but she definitely has a hematoma. What can we do about this?"

"We're hoping it will resorb," the physician answered. "If we try to empty it, the hematoma could rupture, and Ann would bleed out on the table."

Still frustrated and disheartened, Ann was eventually discharged from the hospital. They researched other medical facilities in the U.S. and decided to fly to a cancer center in Utah. Although flying to the mainland was risky, Ann and Don decided it was necessary to seek different treatment.

The difference in her care at the Utah cancer center was remarkable. The physicians at the cancer center reworked her entire treatment plan. "We don't agree with the chemo recipe that you were given," Ann was told. They also replaced the previous stent with a different kind to alleviate the urination problem.

When asked about the hematoma in her stomach, the physician at the cancer center said reassuringly, "We'll take care of that first thing in the morning."

"What time is the surgery?" Ann asked, thinking she was facing a serious operation with a possible bad outcome. She needed to prepare her family and herself.

"Oh, there's no operation. We'll do a CT [computerized tomography] scan and insert a couple of drains. It's an easy procedure," he said reassuringly.

Most importantly, Ann was no longer regarded as the "annoying patient." She was relieved to be treated respectfully by everyone she encountered.

The cancer center's treatment plan called for eight sessions of chemo, three weeks apart. However, Ann didn't handle the chemo very well. She grew weaker, became susceptible to infections, and had trouble walking. After the sixth session, the oncologist told Ann, "We can't give you anymore. If we do, it'll kill you." Fortunately, it was enough, as Ann was now cancer-free.

So, after an eighteen-month recuperation period, including a full regimen of physical therapy, Ann finally recovered. She and Don sold their beloved house in Hawaii and decided to move to Utah to be closer to the cancer center. However, Ann's struggles were not over yet.

In 2010, after a CA 19-9 (cancer antigen) blood test and a CT scan, Ann learned that her cancer had returned—this time in her pancreas. A Whipple procedure was performed, in which most of her pancreas was removed. With the loss of her pancreas, she would need lifelong insulin and enzyme replacement.

Recovery from Whipple surgery was long and difficult. At home one night after the surgery, Ann began to experience severe pain. Her husband said, "Go lie down, and I'll call your surgeon."

"I'm afraid I'll die if I lie down," Ann cried.

Don was unable to reach her surgeon, who was out of the country at a conference. "I'll take you to the emergency room," Don replied.

"No, I don't trust the ER," declared Ann. "Those doctors don't know my case. I'll wait until the morning and see my regular oncologist at the hospital."

It turned out that the pain was due to a bad urinary tract infection, and she was given medication. Her doctor told Ann, "As a cancer center patient here, you can always admit yourself right to the hospital and bypass the emergency room. I'm sorry I forgot to tell you that."

Unfortunately, this wasn't the end of Ann's healthcare journey. In 2014, Ann experienced an aortic aneurysm due to a congenital defect, one that had existed throughout her entire life. Ann remarked, "That's probably why I had limited energy growing up. I thought I was just lazy." She underwent open heart surgery and a subsequent cardiac rehab program.

Despite the series of health issues, Ann has retained her optimistic perspective and has enjoyed the subsequent years of her life. Blessed to have the support of her husband and family, as well as the wonderful care of her local healthcare providers, Ann made a commitment to live fully. She now spends much of her time trying to keep up with her sixteen grandchildren. Ann has traveled with her grandchildren to many countries around the world. In addition, Ann and her husband hold a four-day "cousins summer camp" for all the grandchildren. Despite the many health setbacks, Ann says she has the best life and tries to live thankfully each day.

LESSONS LEARNED

- Ann's health problems continued over several years and involved many different specialists. Because of the disagreement and the confusion that resulted, Ann and Don finally contacted their primary care physician to help coordinate her care. Having someone serve as "the quarterback" is key to avoiding this all-too-common scenario.

- Don was present at each interaction to take notes and to help with the coordination and recollection of instructions.

- Ann was fortunate to have the ability to seek care in another state with healthcare professionals who were knowledgeable, patient-focused, and able to work as a team to coordinate her care, which proved to be critical to her recovery.

- Ann's positive outlook and support from her family continue to be instrumental to her overall health and well-being today.

WHAT YOU NEED TO KNOW

For many patients with serious medical conditions, it is not unusual for a variety of healthcare practitioners, hospitals, and other facilities to be involved. However, with many different specialists involved, there may not be one "quarterback" who has a detailed view of the whole picture and coordinates the ongoing care. Sometimes a patient is given conflicting instructions, making understanding, decision-making, and adherence to the treatment plan confusing and possibly even harmful. Moreover, patients may be given medications without fully understanding whether any current ones are contraindicated or even still necessary. The risk is further increased for someone who has been in the hospital and may be confused due to fear, sleep deprivation, medication, or pain. Incomplete discharge instructions, lack of scheduled follow-up care, and inadequate communication between the hospital, PCP, and/or other care settings (e.g., rehab facility), can also add to the coordination problem.

In the hospital setting, providers from different departments involved in a patient's care may not meet regularly as a team to discuss a specific patient's case. And, although the medical services provided may be documented in the individual hospital's system, a physician may not have consulted with another department's physician to gain a complete understanding of the condition. If, for example, a patient is being seen by physicians in oncology, infectious disease, and plastic surgery, they may not have conferred to create a unified treatment plan. On some occasions, there may be a limited amount of time to resolve any differing opinions and to reach agreement on next steps and the overall course of action. And not infrequently, the patient or family member may not have been included in any discussions at all. Lacking an understanding of medical terminology and having limited communication with the physicians, the patient may be confused about the treatment plan and have little opportunity to ask questions.

Depending on the number of medical professionals involved in a patient's care, this fragmented situation can be even more prevalent in outpatient settings. People often seek care from a variety of healthcare practitioners at individual offices, urgent care facilities, ambulatory centers, and pharmacies, without any one provider or entity knowing about the others. The diagnoses, treatments, and medications are often not documented in a central location or medical record. And the degree of complexity increases for those with multiple problems and/or serious conditions that are inherently complicated, such as cancer.

Coordination via Patient Portals

As mentioned in Chapter 4, your healthcare provider may offer a patient portal, a secure online system that can be used to send and receive messages and store your personal medical record, including lab, radiology, and other test results. This is a good way to coordinate your medical information in one place—if your healthcare providers actually use the portal and all those involved in your care have access to it.

However, if you go to a physician or healthcare facility with a different patient portal, the portals typically do not "talk" to one another, thus adding to the lack of coordination of care. It's not unusual to have two or three separate portals—with different usernames and passwords—that contain distinct medical records specific to a particular provider or health system.

While patient portals can be very beneficial, it is important to ensure the information is accurate and up to date. Do not assume the medical record in one portal is consistent with another and all physicians or healthcare facilities will have your complete medical record.

Coordinating Medications

The profusion of medications, particularly among seniors, is another example of the fragmentation and lack of coordination of care. Multiple practitioners may be prescribing medications without communicating with each other or even knowing about each other. According to the Lown Institute, 42 percent of U.S. adults take five or more medications, and more than 10 percent take ten or more.[1] As new medications are added, the existing ones may not be reduced or eliminated. Frequently, the side effect(s) of one drug leads to a new condition that requires a different medication, and a "prescribing cascade" ensues. Thus, many seniors—and others on a number of medications—continue to take inappropriate, duplicative, or unnecessary medication. Additionally, drug-drug interactions can cause adverse events, or even death. While pharmacies could take a more proactive role in coordinating medications, staffing shortages can make it challenging for them to do so. Often, the focus may be on controlled substances in states in which a tracking database has been established. When it comes to other types of medication, tracking prescriptions across systems, facilities, offices, and states is a complex undertaking for which there may not be sufficient infrastructure in place.

Over-the-counter (OTC) medications, including supplements, are also important to discuss with your healthcare providers in all care settings, both inpatient and outpatient. Some can interact with prescription medications, leading to side effects and/or making them more or less effective. Be sure to include these in the medical record of the portal.

Ensuring Your Care Is Well Coordinated

If you have multiple health conditions and several providers are involved, you cannot assume that your care will be coordinated. Below are steps you can take proactively to help ensure everyone is in the loop and your care is well coordinated:

Make sure you have a primary care practitioner (PCP) and stay connected

We talked about the importance of having someone who knows you and your medical history. Your PCP should be aware when you see any specialists and should be copied on any notes, which should then be added to your medical record. You will need to alert your PCP about any urgent care or emergency room visits so you can receive the appropriate follow-up care in a timely fashion. You will also need to keep them apprised of any new issues and concerns, as well as changes in symptoms, medications, immunizations, allergies, family history, and other healthcare practitioners involved in your care.

Identify the "quarterback"

If you're in the hospital and seeing a variety of practitioners from different departments, ask which one is designated as the "quarterback" to coordinate your care. Ensure this person is aware of all the procedures, test results, and medications involved in your care. If you receive conflicting information or are confused, ask the quarterback to convene the group, reach agreement, address any of your concerns, and communicate the plan in a way you can easily understand.

Become integral to the process

Decisions about your treatment plan and ongoing care should be made with you so your concerns and wishes are heard, understood, and given full consideration. You should understand the options available, along with any associated risks/potential side effects, and be aware if there are any different points of view or opinions. Remember, while you may not be a medical professional, you know your body best. Your comfort level with the ongoing treatment and follow-up care will impact your ability to engage with and adhere to the plan as well as your sense of well-being as you go forward.

Document as much as possible

When seeing multiple healthcare providers over several weeks, months, or even years, it's quite easy to forget what transpired and the instructions you were given. You may be feeling nervous or anxious during a visit with a physician or faced with a major procedure and have difficulty later recalling the exact next steps. If you can bring a trusted family member or friend with you to take notes, it can help tremendously. It is also important for your healthcare provider to document all actions in the medical record at the end of your visit, so it is updated in a timely fashion. Your medical record should be current with all medications, allergies, test results, insurance info, etc. Many hospitals have their own individual systems that include a patient portal so you can see what is written in the medical record. Unfortunately, there is no one universal system among all healthcare facilities or provider offices. So, you'll want to ensure that documentation is captured accurately.

Take advantage of the benefits and programs available through your insurance plan

Some employers and health plans provide navigators who can help you better understand the healthcare system and provide support as you encounter each step in the process. Depending on your situation, case managers and social workers may also be available, particularly if you are hospitalized, are pregnant, have cancer, or have an underlying chronic condition. You may also have second-opinion services available depending on what your employer or insurance plan provides.

Some hospital systems also provide navigation services for patients undergoing care for a complicated condition like cancer. Social workers are often standard resources available during hospitalization and at the time of discharge. They should be involved in helping arrange for any equipment you may need at home. They are knowledgeable of local community and national organizational resources and can help identify facilities for transfer to a subacute or rehab facility. They should also keep your insurance company apprised to help ensure the appropriate approvals are obtained and to reduce the likelihood of issues with insurance claims after discharge.

Take advantage of the patient advocate at the hospital

Most institutions have a patient advocate you can request if you are concerned about your care while hospitalized. This person would be able to have conversations with the myriad individuals involved to help get things on track if you feel uncomfortable doing so yourself.

When new medications are prescribed, ask questions

You will want to know about possible side effects, drug-drug interactions, if meds should be taken with food or on an empty stomach, if alcohol should be avoided, and if there are any contraindications with what you're currently taking. Ask if you still need the current medications, or if you can stop or gradually come off them. Be sure you know what each pill is for and why you're taking it. Update your

EXAMPLES OF TYPES OF CARE COORDINATION[2]

Primary care coordination—". . . some providers have adopted a 'guided primary care' approach. The Guided Care model was developed by a team of researchers at Johns Hopkins University, to respond to the growing challenge of caring for a rapidly aging America. In the Guided Care model, a specially educated, registered nurse (RN) is responsible for patients with multiple chronic conditions. The RN performs an initial assessment on each patient, works directly with the primary care practitioners to develop a care plan, and coordinates specialty care with other providers to ensure that nothing is missed, and the plan is followed."

Acute care coordination—After an emergency has passed and hospital discharge has occurred, acute care coordinators oversee the transition of patient care including scheduling follow-up visits, filling prescriptions, and confirming additional patient instructions. This can impact readmissions and reduce mortality.

Post-acute/long-term care coordination—When patients are also residents in a nursing facility, transitions between levels of care involve changes in medication and care plans. Inadequate care transitions are a big risk for this population. Care coordinators in this setting work with patients and their caregivers to ensure everyone understands the care plan, has proper expectations, and advocates for maintaining the best patient "quality of life" possible.

medical record with the new regimen of medications and be sure to update the records at the pharmacy as well.

Coordination of care is one of the biggest challenges in the U.S. healthcare system. Services can be very fragmented, and it often takes the patient (or the patient's advocate) to ensure all involved are knowledgeable about the care that has been delivered. It should be easier, and perhaps someday it will be. In the meantime, you are in charge of your health and well-being, and ultimately the "buck stops with you." Your life could depend on it!

SO, WHAT CAN YOU DO NOW?

- The human body and the healthcare system are complicated, with lots of opportunities for things to go very well or terribly wrong. Therefore, it is important to be actively engaged in your care every step of the way.

- Educate yourself about your medical condition and make sure you understand the treatment plan.

- Do not assume anyone else sees the entire picture, and be prepared to keep everyone who is involved in your care up to speed and connected. It's up to you to see how the puzzle pieces fit together and to make sure they do.

- Take advantage of all resources available to you, and don't hesitate to seek professional help for any advocacy needs if you can.

CHAPTER 6

Having a Baby

Whether your pregnancy was meticulously planned, medically coaxed, or happened by surprise, one thing is certain—your life will never be the same.

CATHERINE JONES

MARIE'S STORY

Marie and John were married in 2016. Marie was thirty-four, John was forty-four, and both wanted to start having a family right away. John had been married previously for eight years, and he and his first wife were unable to have a baby together, though his ex-wife subsequently got pregnant. Marie and John both underwent a series of fertility tests and confirmed male-factor infertility due to John's very low sperm count. Their fertility doctor said in vitro fertilization (IVF) was their best option and asked if they wanted to use donor sperm, but they were insistent on trying with John's sperm. Given Marie's good fertility health, their doctor's high success rate, and health insurance that covered two rounds of IVF, they proceeded.

After their wedding in April and honeymoon in May, Marie began the egg retrieval process. She produced twenty-one eggs that were then fertilized. Of the twenty-one, fifteen matured to viable embryos. Genetic testing was performed on the embryos and nine were OK—seven girls and two boys. They were graded either A or B and kept frozen.

After a month of recovery and more travels as newlyweds, Marie had a fibroid removed to minimize any IVF problems. This procedure was followed by a few more months of recovery time in preparation for the embryo transfer.

Marie and John decided to have one of the grade A female embryos implanted. It was successful, and on November 5th, Marie learned she was pregnant. She was referred to her regular OB-GYN (obstetrician/gynecologist) to receive the appropriate prenatal care, monitor the pregnancy, and hopefully deliver a healthy baby.

As she had turned thirty-five the month prior, Marie's pregnancy was now considered higher risk. Fellow moms jokingly introduced her to the outdated term *geriatric pregnancy*. This designation made Marie worry, even though her pregnancy seemed to be going smoothly. "Is thirty-five really considered geriatric?" she asked, even though she knew many women were having babies in their late thirties and early forties.

Since this was her first pregnancy, she wasn't sure quite what to expect. With each office visit, Marie rotated through different doctors in the large OB-GYN practice, hardly seeing the same doctor twice. "I don't think my doctor really knows me," Marie told her husband.

At twenty-two weeks, an ultrasound indicated Marie had developed placenta previa, a condition in which the placenta grows too close to the mother's cervix. Marie did not know the potential consequences of placenta previa, and her doctor tried to keep her from worrying by not going into detail about possible excessive bleeding and/or premature birth of the baby. The doctor told Marie, "The placenta will likely move up, but we'll monitor it during the pregnancy." The doctor kept reassuring her it was common, but Marie was still worried. A C-section (Cesarean section) was scheduled for thirty-seven weeks.

But the placenta never moved up. At thirty-six weeks, Marie went for another checkup on a Wednesday afternoon. The placenta previa had evolved to "complete previa," meaning the placenta was fully covering her cervix. She would need to come back in two days to check again and determine whether an immediate C-section was needed. Following another ultrasound on Friday, the doctor called and said, "Everything looks fine. We can wait."

Marie was getting nervous. Why did she need to wait? Wasn't the baby already full term? Was she supposed to wait until something went wrong? Marie was losing confidence in the young doctor. *Maybe she's too inexperienced and I should consult one of the older physicians*, Marie thought to herself. *There's nothing I can do but follow the doctor's orders.*

Monday morning, an hour after John left for work, Marie started bleeding. She began to panic. Is the baby okay? Is the placenta coming out? Will my baby be able to breathe? Her mind raced to the worst-case scenario.

She called her husband, who was in a meeting, then her mother, who was at the hairdresser. "Go to the hospital right now," her mother said. "I will meet you there. I will call John."

To avoid delay, Marie hurried into her car and drove herself to the hospital. With the car's caution lights flashing,

Marie drove very slowly on the shoulder of the highway all the way. She abandoned her car at the emergency room entrance and rushed into the hospital with blood running down her leg. Her mother arrived at the same time, gave Marie's car keys to the guard at the front desk, and asked him to please park the car.

Scared and visibly shaken, Marie was wheeled into the maternity operating room for an emergency C-section. She was given an epidural, a local anesthetic injection, but it didn't go into effect right away. "I can feel everything," Marie cried out. Another injection was administered, which eventually left a numb sensation in her leg for days after the delivery.

Olivia was born via C-section on June 21, 2017, and was immediately moved to the NICU (neonatal intensive care unit). She was having trouble breathing, as her lungs had not fully developed.

Worried about her newborn baby, Marie was discharged from the hospital after three days without Olivia. She returned every day to be with her baby and breastfeed.

Eventually, Olivia's breathing improved, and she was finally allowed to go home. Marie was relieved. Her baby was going to be okay.

In hindsight, Marie knew she had been in a highly emotional state. She should have learned more about placenta previa and asked her doctor what to expect. She should have had a backup emergency plan. She thought everything had been okay, until the bleeding alarmed her and threw her into a panic. "I wish I had been better prepared," Marie reflected.

Eventually, Marie switched to a new OB-GYN practice where she received much more personalized attention and developed the confidence to undergo another pregnancy. In

2018, she underwent a second IVF embryo transfer, this time with a biologically male embryo. Jacob was born vaginally in March 2019, and the experience was much better. She asked questions about the pregnancy and the delivery, so she knew what to expect this time and felt much more comfortable with the new doctor.

Today, Marie and John have two healthy, beautiful children.

LESSONS LEARNED

- Pregnancy and childbirth can be a wonderful but sometimes scary experience. It's critical to learn as much as possible about how to take care of yourself and your baby-to-be, what to expect, and what to do if something unanticipated happens.

- Finding a healthcare practitioner who can provide information and answer questions clearly and completely is critical.

- Fertility issues and multiple births, for example, can present their own set of unique concerns and issues. An understanding of what to expect in these circumstances is vital.

- Having a baby—before, during, and after—can be a highly emotional time. Having an OB-GYN who can also provide comfort and compassion throughout the process and recognize if you need a referral to a behavioral health professional is very important.

- Marie eventually switched to a new practice. Finding a practitioner you can trust and with whom you feel comfortable is crucial.

WHAT YOU NEED TO KNOW

While pregnancy and childbirth can be a joyous event, for many women it can also be frightening and complex, as was the case for Marie. With more reproductive advancements, many women are delaying childbirth to pursue higher education and career opportunities or postponing starting a family until they can afford to do so, particularly given the expense and challenges related to childcare.

Although there is no magic cutoff age, women over thirty-five have traditionally been considered of "advanced maternal age" and may have more difficulty getting pregnant. They may experience a high-risk pregnancy and a higher rate of miscarriage and stillbirth. The rate of gestational diabetes, premature delivery, and low-birth-weight babies is also greater in women ages thirty-five or older who become pregnant.[1]

According to recent statistics on maternal and infant mortality,[2] "the U.S. is the only industrialized nation in the world where maternal mortality is rising." According to the CDC, 861 women died in 2019,[3] and the Commonwealth Fund reports 60,000 women suffer complications of pregnancy each year. As will be discussed in Chapter 11, Black women in the U.S. have a maternal mortality rate that is three to four times higher than their white counterparts, even when education levels and socioeconomic status are the same. Their babies have a mortality rate within the first year that is twice as high. For Latina women, infant and maternal mortality are twice as high compared to white women.

Infertility

Infertility is a clinical state in which a woman is not able to get pregnant after one year of trying, or after six months if a woman is thirty-five or older. In the U.S., 10 percent of men[4] and 10 percent of women are infertile.[5] Overall, one-third of cases of infertility are due to male factors, one-third due to female factors, and one-third due to both male and female factors.[6]

If infertility is a concern, it is important to do your research to find the best physician/infertility clinic for you, including information on the particular method, the success rates, and the cost of services. In vitro fertilization (IVF) and other fertility treatments can be expensive, and they take a big commitment, so you'll want to find what's right for you.

Same-sex couples can face additional hurdles when trying to have a baby.[7] For example, health insurance benefits may not be inclusive, with infertility coverage defined only from the perspective of a heterosexual couple. If using a surrogate, there may also be legal issues regarding parental rights, as in many states the person who gives birth is considered the legal parent. This situation may also come into play for heterosexual couples using a surrogate.

Emotions can run high in couples experiencing infertility. Frustration, disappointment, low self-esteem, anxiety, and depression can result. Combined with the financial pressures of infertility treatment, tensions can become great enough that some relationships do not survive. Seeking help from a medical professional can aid in coping with a difficult situation and getting through with resilience.

Lastly, studies[8] have shown that infertility treatments and conception methods—in vitro fertilization (IVF), intrauterine insemination (IUI), and ovulation drugs—have been associated with a higher incidence of preterm deliveries and low birth weight (LBW) babies, primarily with a higher likelihood of a multiple gestation (more than one baby at a time) pregnancy.

Be Proactive

If possible, it is important to take certain steps in advance of any attempts to become pregnant. Being proactive increases the likelihood of an uncomplicated pregnancy and delivery and reduces the risk of potentially avoidable medical issues for the baby. As mentioned in Chapter 2, good eating habits, regular physical activity, adequate sleep, and stress management are important investments in your health as well as that of your baby-to-come. By maintaining a healthy weight and good control over any underlying health conditions, like diabetes and hypertension, you can better protect yourself and the baby.

Additionally, it is important to be aware of conditions that may impact fertility, pregnancy, and delivery, as well as the baby's health. For example, women with fibroids may have more difficulty becoming pregnant and/or carrying a baby to term. In some instances, addressing the fibroids in advance of pregnancy is a proactive action women can take.

Another proactive measure is genetic testing. Before becoming pregnant, women and their partners can be tested for certain genetic disorders, usually through a blood or saliva sample. While there is no certainty that a baby will inherit the disease, you may want to know if you are a carrier of a genetic abnormality, particularly if it is common among your specific population or community.

SOME INHERITED CONDITIONS THAT GENETIC TESTING CAN DETECT

- Cystic fibrosis—A condition that can progressively damage the lungs and make it harder to breathe

- Fragile X syndrome—A condition more common among males; causes intellectual disabilities and learning challenges

- Sickle cell disease—An inherited blood disorder that causes red blood cells to become crescent shaped, leading to anemia, severe pain, infections, and hospitalization; most often found in the Black population as well as among those of Arab, Greek, Italian, Sardinian, Turkish, Maltese, and southern Asian ancestry

- Tay-Sachs disease—A rare disorder of a missing enzyme that can destroy nerve cells in the brain and spinal cord and lead to early death; more commonly found among Eastern and Central European Jews, as well as certain French Canadians in Quebec, Older Order Amish in Pennsylvania, and Cajuns of Louisiana

- Spinal muscular atrophy—A neurological disorder in which muscles used for movement are weakened and waste away

- Phenylketonuria (PKU)—A metabolic disorder where the body is unable to use an amino acid called *phenylalanine*, which then builds up in the body, and, if the affected person is not on a strict diet, can lead to brain damage

Important note: The FDA (Food and Drug Administration) has issued a warning of potential risks with certain genetic tests that look for genetic abnormalities in a fetus using a sample of blood.[9] The two types of testing in question are non-invasive prenatal screening (NIPS), which may also be called "cell-free DNA tests," and non-invasive prenatal tests (NIPT). The FDA has identified three potential risks: false results, inappropriate use, and inaccurate interpretation of results. The FDA recommends seeking the help of a genetic counselor to discuss risks and benefits before making a decision regarding a pregnancy based on the results of these tests. In some cases, additional testing may be warranted or advisable.

Prenatal Care

Access to prenatal care is key to a successful pregnancy and healthy baby. Optimally, it includes early and regular visits to the OB-GYN, folic acid supplements (to reduce the risk of neurological disorders related to malformations of the spinal cord, such as spina bifida), prenatal testing, and certain vaccinations.

It is important to ask questions throughout the course of the pregnancy. For example, certain vaccines are recommended, and others should be postponed. Tobacco, e-cigarette/vaping, alcohol, or illicit drug use increases the risk of a premature delivery, miscarriage, birth defects, sudden infant death syndrome (SIDS), and fetal alcohol syndrome. It is important to let your healthcare practitioner know of any addictions so precautions can be taken to help protect your baby and to get the help you need.

Open communication and a true partnership with your physician are critical, as we discussed in Chapter 4.

Knowing what to expect and how to take care of yourself to support the baby's growth and development during pregnancy are vital to the delivery of a healthy baby. Don't be afraid to ask questions and share any concerns, so you become more secure in your knowledge and receive the care you need.

If you have insurance, some health plans, including Medicaid, provide educational programs to support and help you navigate throughout the pregnancy as well as following delivery. For those with complicated, high-risk pregnancies, a case manager may also be available for support.

Maternity Complications

Up to 28 percent of pregnant women experience complications. The impact of some may be limited to the time of the pregnancy itself, while others may have an impact on the future health of the mother and/or baby. Below are the more common situations that may arise. In addition to prenatal care and a healthy lifestyle, if you have had a prior high-risk pregnancy or if you develop complications, you may well need to be followed by an OB who specializes in high-risk pregnancies.

Miscarriage

Also known as spontaneous abortion, miscarriage is the loss of a known pregnancy before the twentieth week. Ten to twenty percent of pregnancies end in a miscarriage,[10] but the actual rate may be higher because many miscarriages happen before a woman knows she is pregnant.

Risk factors for miscarriage include an older maternal age (particularly after age forty), prior history of miscarriage, smoking and/or use of alcohol and/or illicit drugs, underlying medical conditions, particularly if they are not well managed, anatomical issues with the uterus or cervix, being overweight or obese, and, on rare occasions, certain prenatal testing. However, many miscarriages are unrelated to any parental factors but rather a situation in which the fetus is not developing properly.

Symptoms of a miscarriage can include vaginal bleeding, cramping, stomach/back pain, or a passing of tissue and gush of fluid from the vagina. If you think you are experiencing a miscarriage, the general guidance is to contact your physician right away and go to the emergency room immediately if you are unable to connect promptly.

Miscarriage can be a devastating experience for parents. Unfortunately, it is a topic that is often not discussed by those in pain and mourning the loss. Family and friends are often not sure what to say or do. Seeking help and support can be a critical part of the healing process.

Anemia

Anemia is common during pregnancy (up to 18 percent of women are anemic) and is one of the reasons women are prescribed prenatal vitamins. The risk of anemia is greater in a multiple gestation or teen pregnancy, when suffering from severe vomiting during pregnancy, being anemic prior to being pregnant, or having a diet with insufficient intake of iron.

A recent study[11] indicates moderate to severe anemia increases the risk of premature delivery, a low birth weight baby, stillbirth, maternal shock, severe postpartum hemorrhage, ICU admission, postpartum depression, maternal death, fetal malformation, and developmental delays.

Gestational diabetes

Seven percent of pregnant women develop gestational diabetes. At greater risk are women of color, being overweight/obese, having high blood pressure or heart disease, personal or family history of diabetes or prediabetes, or having polycystic ovary syndrome (PCOS).[12] You can expect to be tested at twenty-four to twenty-eight weeks of your pregnancy.

Gestational diabetes increases the risk of:

- Stillbirth (death of a baby after twenty weeks of pregnancy)
- Having a baby weighing more than eight pounds, which can lead to an increased risk of a C-section to prevent the baby's shoulders from getting stuck during delivery and other birth injuries
- Breathing problems, jaundice, and/or low blood sugar in the baby
- Diabetes and/or obesity in mother and baby later in life

Hyperemesis gravidarum

Hyperemesis gravidarum (HG) is excessive vomiting severe enough to disrupt day-to-day life and is seen in less than 3 percent of pregnancies. It usually starts between the fourth and sixth weeks of pregnancy, reaches its apex between the ninth and thirteenth weeks, and gets better by week twenty. Women may become dehydrated enough to require hospitalization, may lose weight (5 percent or more weight loss is common), may develop kidney and electrolyte problems, may need to receive nutrition by vein, and may require bed rest. 20 percent of women with HG will continue to have problems after week twenty.

Risk factors for HG include a history of motion sickness and a prior episode of hyperemesis gravidarum.

Preeclampsia

Guidelines from the American College of Obstetricians and Gynecologists (ACOG)[13] define preeclampsia as the development of persistent high blood pressure that arises during pregnancy after week 20. It is associated with high levels of protein in the urine or decreased blood platelets, headaches, visual disturbances, problems with the liver or kidneys, or fluid in the lungs.

Preeclampsia develops in 4 percent of pregnancies in the U.S. Risk factors for preeclampsia include: first pregnancy; age thirty-five or older; personal or family history of preeclampsia; those with kidney disease, diabetes, or an autoimmune condition; obesity; multiple gestation pregnancy; pregnancy via IVF; being Black; having a low-income status; and a span of ten years or more between pregnancies. If preeclampsia is not successfully treated medically, then delivery of the baby and placenta is indicated.

Placenta previa

Placenta previa occurs when the placenta partially or completely covers the cervix. It occurs in up to 15 percent of pregnancies. The risk is increased in women with fibroids or those with uterine scarring from prior surgery. Placenta previa requires delivery by C-section, usually two to four weeks before the due date.

Perinatal depression

Perinatal depression can occur during pregnancy and can continue up to one year after delivery. Symptoms include extreme sadness, anxiety, and fatigue. Although postpartum depression may be more commonly known, up to 7 percent of women experience depression before they give birth. Risk factors for perinatal depression include extreme stress or anxiety, a prior history of depression, an unintended pregnancy, insufficient support, domestic abuse, and preexisting depression prior to pregnancy.

Midwives and Doulas

For low-risk pregnancies, some women decide to use a midwife rather than an obstetrician. A midwife is a trained healthcare professional who can provide prenatal care and deliver a baby in or outside of a hospital—for example, at home or at a birthing center. A certified midwife is trained to provide a more natural, vaginal birth in a more holistic environment. While some may also work with an obstetrician, a midwife is often able to spend more time getting to know the mother/couple and addressing their needs during the pregnancy. However, if the pregnancy is high risk—if there are health complications or multiple births—the expertise needed (as well as any surgery that might need to be performed) is typically not within the scope of services a midwife is trained or licensed to provide.

Though not licensed to provide medical treatment, a doula provides physical and emotional comfort and support during the pregnancy and delivery and afterward. By acting as birthing coaches, doulas can assist with breathing and relaxation techniques and help make childbirth a less frightening and more comfortable experience. After delivery, a doula can support the new mother in adjusting to the new baby, helping with breastfeeding, and allowing her to rest.

You will want to check your insurance to see whether the costs for a midwife or a doula are covered. Some plans may cover a midwife's fees only if the birth is performed in a hospital.

Certification and availability of midwives and doulas vary from state to state. If you are having a low-risk pregnancy, your physician or local hospital may have recommendations for such services. Many OB practices also include midwives. The National Association of Certified Professional Midwives (NACPM) may be a good place to learn more. And if you are interested in having the assistance of a doula for your birth experience, DONA International (previously Doulas of North America) provides a database of certified doulas.

Vaginal Birth and C-Section

About two out of three babies in the United States are born via vaginal delivery, according to the National Center for Health Statistics.[14] Although the mother may incur more pain during vaginal delivery than during a C-section, vaginal births avoid the risk of major surgery and reduce the length of the hospital stay following delivery, which is typically twenty-four to forty-eight hours.

The C-section rate has been increasing in the U.S. and may vary from one part of the country to another, from state to state, and even from hospital to hospital. The rate of low-risk C-sections is higher in Black women compared to white women and Latinas[15] and is also higher in women forty or older.

Although a Cesarean section is generally considered safe, it is still major surgery, has a longer recovery period, and does carry more risk. The usual medical indications for a C-section are conditions or complications that are life threatening to the mother and/or the baby. If you have had a Cesarean birth with your first child, it will be important to ask your obstetrician about a VBAC (vaginal birth after Cesarean) for subsequent births.

The current U.S. rate of repeat C-sections after the first one is greater than 90 percent.[16] However, advances have been made that enable 60 to 80 percent of women to deliver vaginally in future pregnancies following a C-section (depending on the reason a C-section was initially needed).[17]

Regardless of which method of delivery is performed, learn as much as possible about your options, engage in a discussion with your obstetrician, and advocate for what you want—to make the most informed choice.

Postpartum: The "Fourth Trimester"

Regardless of whether the delivery is easy or difficult, it takes time for a woman to recover both physically and mentally from giving birth. Caring for a newborn can be overwhelming, particularly for first-time moms. While the first few months are an important time for bonding, this period is frequently characterized by sleep deprivation, struggles with breastfeeding, and fatigue. In recognition of these challenges, the twelve weeks following delivery are often called the "fourth trimester."

It typically takes at least six to eight weeks for the body to heal, depending on whether the woman had a vaginal delivery or a C-section, and rest is essential for the healing to occur. Women may experience hormonal changes, perhaps resulting in hair loss and emotional volatility. If a partner is in the picture, that person may experience feelings of isolation and jealousy, as the mother and baby become the focus of attention. And if there's little support from family, friends, or home health services, new parents may find it difficult to eat well, rest, and take care of themselves.

Your physician should make you aware of any possible signs of complications that could be life threatening, such as excessive pain, bleeding, or signs of infection, and should provide instructions regarding the steps to take in an emergency. You should also be given instructions about physical activity, nutrition, and sexual activity.

Some women may feel sad or blue after giving birth due to fatigue, stress, and feelings of inadequacy in taking care of a newborn, particularly if the infant only sleeps in "micro naps" and/or cries a lot. Hormonal changes may also contribute to these feelings. In some women these feelings progress to postpartum depression, which is officially defined as major depression that begins within four weeks after delivery and is seen in up to 14 percent of women.[18]

Depression can make it harder to take care of yourself and your baby. It is important to take your feelings seriously, to talk to your physician, and to seek mental health resources in your area, which might include virtual options. If you have insurance coverage, it will also be beneficial to find out what resources may be available through your health plan, including EAP (employee assistance program) services.

The Cost of Having a Baby

Having a baby is expensive. The cost varies by state and depends on whether you have a vaginal or a C-section delivery, where you give birth (in a hospital, birthing center, or home), if you experience any complications, and if you have insurance or not. The average cost of a complication-free vaginal delivery in the United States in 2020 was $10,808.[19] The average cost of a low-risk C-section without complication was much higher, at $22,646.[20] Your out-of-pocket cost will depend on your coinsurance/co-pay, and deductible if you have insurance (see Chapter 11), or the fees charged by your provider and the facility if you do not.

If you factor in the costs of prenatal care—including doctor visits, birthing classes, vitamins, ultrasound, fetal DNA testing, amniocentesis, and other screenings—as well as follow-up postpartum care, the costs can soar. And these costs are even greater if there are complications with "maternal co-morbidities" (chronic medical conditions such as obesity, diabetes, etc.).[21] Of course, the longer you and the baby stay in the hospital, the more expensive it becomes. And if there are fertility problems in conceiving a child, and you choose to have a baby by adoption, by in vitro fertilization, or with a surrogate, you may spend as much as $40,000 or more, per child.[22]

The U.S. is behind many other industrialized countries in the world when it comes to paying for time off for parents after the delivery and covering the subsequent costs of day care or pre-K classes.

At the time of this publication, if you have worked for a company for at least twelve months, have worked at least 1,250 hours over the past twelve months, and are at a location with fifty or more employees within seventy-five miles, you may be eligible for the Family Medical Leave Act (FMLA). This federal law provides up to twelve weeks of "unpaid, job-protected leave per year" for the birth and care of a newborn child. It also allows you to keep your health benefits during your time off from work, as long as you pay your health insurance premiums during that period.

Your company may offer an additional benefit of paternity/partner leave for spouses/partners as well. Depending on your employer, the amount of time off for maternity leave is usually longer for the parent who had the baby or is the primary caregiver; in other words, maternity leave is typically longer than paternity leave.

As is the case with healthcare in general, if you're planning to have a baby, having health insurance can impact not only your health and well-being but that of your baby. Be aware of what your insurance plan will cover. You will also want to check with your employer regarding your eligibility for FMLA and how to pay your health insurance premiums on time, so your coverage doesn't lapse.

Every pregnancy journey is unique. Some are easy and joyful, while others are complicated and may involve loss, grief, and mourning. Planning in advance, practicing healthy lifestyle habits, educating yourself about what to expect and do, and selecting an experienced healthcare practice/practitioner you trust, can maximize the chances of a healthy pregnancy and delivery of a healthy baby.

SO, WHAT CAN YOU DO NOW?

- Having a baby, or losing one, will change your life forever. Living a healthy lifestyle even before you become pregnant and then taking good care of yourself, physically and mentally, during the prenatal period maximizes the likelihood of an uncomplicated pregnancy and delivering a healthy baby.

- Educate yourself, take prenatal classes, and make sure you are under the care of a clinician who can advise you regarding the steps to take for a healthy pregnancy.

- If you have preexisting chronic conditions, it is important to manage them optimally to minimize the risk of a negative impact on you or your baby.

- If you have had complications during a prior pregnancy or suffered a miscarriage or still birth, you may need an OB-GYN who specializes in high-risk pregnancies.

- Ask about your options for the setting in which you deliver your baby.

- Advocate for yourself as needed throughout your pregnancy and the postpartum period.

CHAPTER 7

Deciding Where to Go When a Medical Need Arises

We have really good data that show when you take patients and you really inform them about their choices, patients make more frugal choices. They pick more efficient choices than the health care system does.

DONALD BERWICK, MD

CLIFTON'S STORY

As the COVID-19 pandemic was beginning to spread across the U.S. in early 2020, Americans were slowly learning about the symptoms, its virulence, and the most effective ways to treat the illness. With limited testing, insufficient supplies of protective gear, and overwhelmed emergency rooms and ICUs, healthcare workers faced enormous risks.

In early April 2020, Clifton, a sixty-one-year-old x-ray technologist, began to feel tired and developed a mild cough. He took a sick day on a Friday, thinking he had a bad cold. By Monday, he developed a slight fever and grew even more lethargic. Needing a doctor's note to stay home for a few more days and given his history of asthma, Clifton called his pulmonary specialist for an appointment. His regular pulmonary physician was out of town, so the on-call doctor proceeded to do a chest x-ray. It showed that Clifton's lungs were clear, and, providing the note to excuse him from work, told him he probably just had bronchitis.

Returning home, Clifton stayed in bed and slept throughout the next several days. *This must be the flu*, he thought. His appetite decreased, his fever rose, and the fatigue worsened. Clifton's wife and adult child became increasingly worried. They called Clifton's primary care physician, who told them to take Clifton to the hospital. To expedite the check-in process at the emergency room, they used the local hospital's online web portal and described his symptoms. At the emergency room, Clifton was tested for the coronavirus and was told it would take about a week to get the results. He was sent back home.

Within the next twenty-four to forty-eight hours, Clifton's fever rose to 104 degrees, his appetite disappeared, and the cough persisted. He fell asleep and woke up suddenly crying out, "I can't breathe!" With the help of his wife and adult child, Clifton hobbled to the bathroom sink, where he expelled bloody sputum. He was experiencing shortness of breath and beginning to hallucinate.

He's dying, his wife anxiously thought, and called the hospital to dispatch an ambulance. The call was forwarded to a triage nurse with the emergency room department. "Is the sputum frothy?" she asked, not certain that his condition was serious enough for an emergency room visit.

Clifton's wife refused to wait. His wife and adult child checked in again online, insisting that an ambulance arrive. They accompanied Clifton to the hospital's emergency room a second time. While Clifton was being examined, his wife called Clifton's primary care physician again. "Don't let him leave the hospital without a chest x-ray," the PCP replied.

After insisting on the chest x-ray, they learned Clifton had developed pneumonia. He was moved to a small, closet-like room, in the COVID-19 section of the emergency department. His oxygen saturation level had become dangerously low at 83 to 85 percent. In addition to administering oxygen, they started an IV to treat his dehydration. His family members could enter the room one at a time, but no other visitors were allowed. A second COVID-19 test was taken, and the positive result came back in two days.

After two days in isolation, Clifton was moved to the ICU. His oxygen tube was replaced with a face mask, and all his vital functions were monitored. He was given diuretics to reduce the fluid in his lungs and antibiotics to treat the pneumonia. For eight days, Clifton could barely move. He essentially only slept and urinated. No one was allowed to see him.

Eventually, the medication started working, and his oxygen level began to increase. He had lost thirty pounds within a short span of time.

After ten days, Clifton was relocated to the step-down unit and began to feel better. Still a bit shaky, he was determined to leave and recover at home. Although the nurses were wonderful, he knew they were afraid of him. He could sense their fear of contracting the virus themselves.

Clifton spent the next few weeks at home, slowly regaining his appetite and his strength. He was worried about how to pay for the medical expenses and wondered about the back pay he missed during the past month, as his sick leave had run out. Fortunately, his employer had put him on administrative leave, and he never missed a paycheck.

He took a COVID-19 antibody test, and it was positive. His wife and adult child also tested positive but experienced only mild symptoms for a few days. All the testing was administered at no charge to him and his family.

Back at work, a whole new culture of COVID-19 awareness had developed, and mandates to wear masks, gloves, and protective gear had been instituted. Clifton knew some of his coworkers were afraid for him to come back, thinking he might still be contagious. He was afraid they would run and hide as soon as he returned to work—and some did.

Checking in again with his primary care physician, Clifton was told to ask for a "reasonable accommodation" at work, as mandated by the Americans with Disabilities Act. He needed to be able to recover gradually, allowing his strength and body weight to improve.

Eventually, Clifton returned to work on a reduced schedule. However, his anxiety continued, and he had nightmares about his experience. He would wake up at night thinking he was still in the hospital. He could still remember the curled-up position of his body and the nauseating smell of the oxygen and hand sanitizer. "This anxiety must be what PTSD is like," he thought. At work, he was invited to join a support group to talk about his experience. The support group proved to be therapeutic; talking to others helped. He also appreciated that his friends reached out to him on Facebook, sending caring thoughts and best wishes. And gradually, Clifton grew more relaxed.

He began walking a little farther each day, eventually going the 1.2 miles on foot from his home to his workplace. Finally, he was strong enough to ride his bike to work again. As of this writing, Clifton and his family are well. They are grateful to have survived this ordeal when so many others were not as fortunate.

LESSONS LEARNED

- Clifton survived his bout with COVID-19 in large part due to the persistence and advocacy of his wife and adult child. They saw his health deteriorating and trusted their instincts to take him to the hospital. Even though he was initially sent home from the emergency room, they persevered.

- It's often hard to know what to do when a medical event occurs. Listening to your primary care physician can be crucial. The PCP's demand for another chest x-ray proved to be lifesaving.

- Even after his physical recovery, Clifton realized his mental and emotional health had been affected. Seeking help from a counselor, a support group, or other type of therapy can be valuable in getting back to your life.

WHAT YOU NEED TO KNOW

When we feel sick, many of us wonder whether we should seek medical attention right away or wait to see if we get better on our own. Doctor and emergency room visits can be expensive and time-consuming, and often we are not sure how critical the medical condition is.

If you are seeking medical attention, there may be several options available depending on the resources in your geographic area and the severity and urgency of your condition.

24-Hour Nurse Line

If you are unsure whether your symptoms are serious enough to seek medical attention, a twenty-four-hour nurse line may be your first option. Many insurance plans provide an online chat feature or free phone line with an experienced registered nurse who can discuss your medical condition and concerns and provide advice on what to do and where to go. During the pandemic, COVID-19 hotlines were set up to respond to patient concerns. In addition, mental health resources, including a suicide prevention hotline, may be available to provide confidential support for you and your loved ones.

Your Healthcare Practitioner/Doctor's Office

We talked about the importance of establishing a relationship with a primary care practitioner before you are sick, so there is someone who knows you and your medical history. If you have a chronic condition, your primary care practitioner will have a record of your medications and will know the specialists you have seen. If the office is closed, most have an emergency number so someone on call can be reached. Depending on the severity of the condition, your doctor can help advise you about where to go and can coordinate your care with the hospital or other healthcare practitioner.

Federally Qualified Health Centers (FQHCs)

A Federally Qualified Health Center (FQHC) is "a community-based outpatient clinic that provides comprehensive primary care services to a designated Medically Underserved Area (MUA) or Medically Underserved Population (MUP). . . . The comprehensive services of an FQHC can include preventive care, dental care, chronic disease management, mental health and substance abuse, or hospital and specialty care.... A variety of health care providers such as physicians, physician assistants, dentists, certified nurse-midwives, clinical psychologists, clinical social workers, and pharmacists can provide services at an FQHC."[1]

They often have a variety of services under one roof and can help coordinate your care. And for those in rural areas, which often have the same health and healthcare system issues as the poor in underserved areas of cities, the Health Resources and Services Administration (HRSA) has resources that may help.

Telemedicine/Telehealth (Virtual Care)

The recent pandemic has resulted in a rapid increase in the availability of technology-enabled services that provide the ability to visit with a healthcare provider by using your smartphone or computer. If you are frequently on the road for work or have a tightly regulated work schedule, or if traveling to the provider's office is difficult or inconvenient, you may be able to set up a telemedicine visit to discuss your concerns, explore treatment options, and even get prescriptions for medications if needed. Mental health services are also available virtually. However, if you need an in-person physical examination, or if you have an urgent situation, this approach is not medically appropriate. You will want to get information from the healthcare provider's office or telehealth service, in advance of your appointment, so the virtual visit goes smoothly.

Walk-in Clinics/Retail Clinics versus Urgent Care

In the case of a minor illness or injury—a cut or a minor burn; sprain of an ankle, knee, or shoulder; or a bad cold or the flu, ear infection, strep throat, or pink eye—you may not be able to get an appointment with your physician quickly, or it may be inconvenient to get to the doctor's office. Although you may be able to schedule an appointment, most retail clinics and urgent care centers provide services to those who walk in without one. A retail clinic, though not generally open twenty-four hours a day, typically treats uncomplicated health issues (e.g., cold or flu), and is usually staffed by a nurse practitioner or physician assistant.

An urgent care center is designed to address more complex problems or injuries that may require a workup, perhaps with x-rays, blood tests, or simple stitching. Many will be open 24/7 and have a team that includes a physician and more than one exam room. Depending on the severity of your problem, urgent care centers may be an appropriate alternative due to their convenient location, extended hours, and generally lower costs when compared to the same services provided in an emergency room. And, depending on the time and number of patients, you may be able to see a doctor much sooner than you could see your own doctor. However, these places supplement your care, and do not take the place of your primary care physician, whom you would want to see for follow-up and ongoing care. Urgent care centers and walk-in clinics are not appropriate for severe, life-threatening injuries or illnesses or for primary care.

It's important to remember that urgent care centers are not governed by the same laws as emergency rooms, and they are not required to see and stabilize a patient like an emergency room must do. One example is patients who have been in a car accident. Sometimes urgent care centers will not accept and provide care to a patient because they are not adequately equipped to address the injuries that have been sustained. In other instances, they may refer the patient to an emergency room, particularly if they are in the same health system, for financial reasons. Financial margins can be thin for urgent care centers, and the process of getting reimbursement related to auto insurance can be prolonged. Unfortunately, some patients may end up paying the cost of an urgent care visit just to find out they need additional care in the emergency room, in which case they may be stuck with two bills.[2]

Ambulatory care center

If you need testing, imaging, or outpatient surgery, an ambulatory care center may be an appropriate setting. While they may be affiliated with a hospital, health system, or medical group, ambulatory care centers offer medical services when an inpatient setting and the additional equipment, specialized support, and backup are not required. Ambulatory surgery centers may handle a variety of procedures such as tonsillectomies, cataract surgery, biopsies, and knee replacement surgery that may not require extended observation and an overnight stay. In addition to potentially being more convenient than a hospital, the cost of services delivered in a less acute care setting is typically far less, which is important when it comes to any co-pays or coinsurance involved in your health insurance, or if you have no coverage and must pay for all the expenses incurred.

Some ambulatory care centers are part of a hospital/health system and others may be stand-alone and unaffiliated. The latter will usually be less expensive than those that may include administrative and other facility fees related to the overhead expenses of the hospital or health system.

Hospital Emergency Room

In a normal year, approximately 145 million people visit an emergency room. With the outbreak of the pandemic, some people were afraid to go to emergency rooms, even though doctors, nurses, and administrators were working diligently to implement protocols to minimize the spread of the virus. However, if a situation is or could be life threatening—perhaps a severe trauma, burn, or injury; a possible stroke or

OBSERVATION STAY

There is a category of care known as an "observation stay." It is what its name implies. When a patient is evaluated in the ER, it is not always clear if they are ill enough to require hospitalization, or if care in the ER will be sufficient to allow for discharge. A patient may be observed in the ER or in another part of the hospital on a regular patient floor. An observation stay is considered outpatient, although you may end up staying for more than one day and overnight. In such situations, the patient can receive services and be watched for up to forty-eight hours. If a patient is not ready for discharge at the end of forty-eight hours, then admission to the hospital as an inpatient would occur.

To avoid an unpleasant surprise when a bill is received, it is important to ask if you are considered to be in observation or a regular ER visit. Depending on the type of insurance you have, the portion of the charges for which you will be responsible may be much higher than expected and can be greater than for an inpatient admission.[3]

heart attack, a loss of consciousness, persistent pain, and/or difficulty breathing—you should call 911 to get to an emergency room immediately. While emergency room visits are far more costly than outpatient care settings, emergency room providers are specially trained to act quickly and save lives. If you do not have health insurance, the emergency room cannot deny essential lifesaving services. However, you will be billed for all medical services provided. Hospital emergency rooms should not be used for primary care or minor ailments that would be better addressed by a primary care practitioner or urgent care facility and at far lower cost to you.

In some parts of the country, a stand-alone ER may be available. A stand-alone ER is a licensed facility that provides emergency care but is structurally a separate and distinct entity from a hospital. There are two types: (1) a hospital outpatient department (HOPD) and (2) an independent freestanding emergency center (IFEC). It is important to know that an IFEC can be owned and operated by an individual or private entity.

You should be aware that, although some of these facilities may feel more like an outpatient facility or urgent care clinic when you arrive, the fees are similar or sometimes even higher than an ER located inside a hospital. If an HOPD accepts Medicare or Medicaid, it must follow the same rules and regulations as a regular ER. If it does not, it is subject to the rules and regulations of the state, which means they may vary depending on your location.

At the current time, the Centers for Medicare and Medicaid Services do not recognize IFECs as emergency rooms, and therefore some components of care are not reimbursed, in which case many of the charges will be your sole responsibility. Some commercial health plans offered through employers do not cover care delivered in a stand-alone ER or include these facilities in their network, especially if a regular in-hospital ER is available.

Inpatient (Hospital)

Admission to a hospital is indicated when one suffers a health event that cannot be managed on an outpatient basis. Examples include a heart attack, stroke, car accident with serious injuries, appendicitis, and severe COVID-19. Within a hospital there are several levels of care: regular floor, a step-down unit, and the ICU (intensive care unit—medical, surgical, neonatal, etc.). Patients on a regular unit do not require as intense or complicated care as those in a step-down unit or ICU.

Centers of Excellence (COE)

A separate department of a hospital or a stand-alone facility may create a Center of Excellence (COE) that brings together an interdisciplinary team of healthcare specialists and sometimes researchers, focused on a specific medical condition, such as cancer or cardiovascular care, or a particular procedure, such as heart valve replacement. Through special expertise, coordination of care, best practices, and a high volume of patients, COEs can provide higher quality care and better clinical outcomes, thereby also lowering the cost of care. Depending on the condition or procedure, the COE team will often follow care pathways, which are protocols for managing patient care. The care pathways are designed to reduce any medically unsubstantiated variations in care delivery, thereby increasing quality and cost-efficiency. COEs are often at the forefront of innovation.

There are certain requirements and characteristics involved in being designated a COE. Once you have identified or have been referred to a COE, check to make sure these requirements have been met. It is also important to know that a COE designation is not permanent. For example, if key surgeons leave the team, then COE performance may suffer and may no longer make the grade.

If you have a chronic or unusual medical condition and may be having limited success with your current treatment plan, you may want to do some research to find a Center of Excellence. There are several potential ways to access a COE:

- Your health insurer may have information to share. In fact, in some instances, your insurer may require you to use a COE for certain conditions or procedures. Your co-pay or coinsurance may be lower or waived if you use one. Some common areas for a COE include transplants, joint replacements, and bariatric surgery.

- Your employer may provide information. In some instances, you may be required to use one for certain procedures or conditions or to provide additional support. For example, Walmart has an expansive program for its employees.[4]

- Ask your primary care practitioner or specialist for a recommendation. You may want to seek a second opinion at a COE.

Assessing the situation when a medical issue arises requires alertness and quick decision-making. You know your own body best. It is better to err on the side of caution and seek medical guidance if you are concerned and not sure what to do. Depending on your medical issue, taking prompt action may be critical to obtaining the proper treatment before a health condition worsens, becomes life threatening, or the number of care options available to you shrinks.

SO, WHAT CAN YOU DO NOW?

- In medicine, it is important to be at the right place at the right time to receive the most appropriate care. The right place may help reduce the high cost of medical bills and out-of-pocket expenses, such as going to the emergency room when the condition could have been handled in an urgent care setting or a doctor's office. On the other hand, going to an urgent care center with symptoms of a heart attack may put your life in jeopardy if you delay being treated in a place staffed and equipped to handle such a time-critical situation. So, it's important to find out about the different healthcare settings and facilities in your area and the medical services they offer.

- Take time to review your health plan coverage and your financial responsibility for each setting, for example, co-pay/coinsurance and deductible.

- Select the best place for your health issue, depending on the urgency and degree of severity. Your PCP should be able to provide guidance.

CHAPTER 8

Maintaining Your Emotional Health

Anything that's human is mentionable, and anything that is mentionable can be more manageable. When we can talk about our feelings, they become less overwhelming, less upsetting, and less scary.

FRED ROGERS

DIRK'S STORY

In February 2011, Dirk, a healthy, six-foot five, fifty-year-old marketing executive, traveled to Colorado on a ski vacation with his wife, Lucy, along with eight friends, one of whom was a physician. After one morning run, his wife decided to quit early and return to the hotel. Dirk and his friends headed up the mountain to ski the expert slopes. As he got off the ski lift at the top of the mountain, Dirk suddenly experienced what felt like a sharp lightning bolt of pain from the front of his throat to his lower back. Bent over his ski poles, Dirk moaned to his friends, "I think I am having some sort of altitude event." Very much in pain, he managed to ski down the mountain to meet his wife, determined to lie down at the hotel. But the pain continued, and he could not rest. They set off quickly to the emergency room at the small clinic in the ski town.

Ashen and in pain, Dirk could see the look of serious concern on the faces of the clinic's practitioners. After a CT scan, the emergency room physician told Dirk that he had an aortic dissection, a spiral tear inside his aorta from the top of his heart down to his legs.

"You are lucky to be alive," the clinic doctor told him. "We're helicoptering you to a larger hospital in Grand Junction." Dirk began to panic and asked his wife to call their physician friend Bill, who had not been skiing with Dirk earlier. Bill arrived quickly at the clinic and confirmed the diagnosis. "This is really happening," his friend urgently advised. "They seem to know what they are doing. I would trust their advice. Go now." *How fortunate,* Dirk thought, *to have a trusted friend and physician there at the right time.*

During the helicopter ride to Grand Junction, Dirk observed the magnificent sunset blazing in the sky out the window. The trip seemed surreal, and, like a sightseeing tourist, he managed to remain calm to admire the view.

Landing on the hospital roof, the emergency team raced to the helicopter. *It's like a TV show,* Dirk thought. They immediately began readying him for surgery. When the surgeon explained the high risk of open-heart surgery, Dirk insisted, "I need to talk to my kids first." Lucy called and miraculously managed to get them both on the phone. Calling the two boys, ages twenty and twenty-four, usually meant leaving a message and waiting for a call back. But on this night, they both picked up, and Dirk was able to speak to them briefly before being whisked into the operating room.

Dirk awoke from surgery with five tubes emanating from his body and one tube down his throat. He remained in the hospital at Grand Junction for the next six weeks. During that time, his kidneys began to fail, he developed complications with two bouts of pneumonia, and he suffered through a painful bout of pancreatitis. A few days after the initial surgery, he experienced an irrational panic, telling his wife, "I have to get out of here." Lucy responded with calm reassurance, "No, this is a great place, and you're in good hands."

Aware of the severity of her husband's condition, Lucy provided critical hope and support. When Dirk told her that he might "still be taken," she told him, "This only works if we are together." Lucy's quiet comfort and communication of confidence were exactly what Dirk needed.

Dirk relaxed and learned to accept his present situation. By relinquishing control and releasing his resistance, Dirk began to put his trust in the nurses and doctors at the hospital and grew more at peace. He began talking with the healthcare workers, asking them questions to learn about them as people; he built a personal rapport with each one. Dirk was grateful for every person that came into his room every day and expressed appreciation for their care. "Thank you," he said to everyone, including the aides that came to clean his room and the ones who woke him up in the middle of the night to draw blood.

"People aren't always nice like you," they replied, buoying his spirits. Dirk believed that by focusing on others, he would be in a relaxed "state of grace" and greater healing could follow.

While he was not fully recovered, the doctors decided he was well enough to travel home to the East Coast, with the goal of getting him to lower altitude. But within two days of being home, Dirk began coughing blood. On the third day, he was admitted to the pulmonary ICU at his local hospital, where he spent the next two weeks. While there, Dirk continued his refusal to fight against his current condition and focused his attention instead on healing. Adopting a spiritual perspective, Dirk thought about what Lucy had said to him: "You were flying high like an eagle before. Now you must become the bear—grounded yet still powerful." *It's not about me*, Dirk reminded himself. *It's about staying strong for my family.*

After leaving the hospital, Dirk worked hard at recovery. After nine months, he finally felt some semblance of normal. But in the following few years, the doctors discovered Dirk's aorta had begun to fail, and his life was at risk again. In September 2014, Dirk had a second heart surgery. Dreading another procedure, Dirk asked for his youngest son, Nathaniel, to accompany him and his wife on the two-day drive to the hospital. "Nathaniel makes me laugh," Dirk said. "He has a lightness of being and helps me stay positive."

During this second surgery, the aortic arch was replaced with a Dacron tube and a mechanical valve was implanted in his heart. Before and after the surgery, Dirk continued to converse on a personal level with the healthcare workers, willingly turning over the control of his care to them. "This ability to relinquish control created a sense of equanimity," Dirk reflected, "and allowed me to reduce stress and stay calm." The second surgery was successful, and, after another extended period of convalescence at home, Dirk resumed his daily life.

However, more procedures were still to come. In June 2016, Dirk suddenly needed an emergency appendectomy. Facing yet another surgery, Dirk consciously endeavored to resume his state of equanimity, a strategy that again helped him through an unexpected health event.

A year or so after recovering from this third surgery, Dirk's hip began to fail, and he was told he would need a hip replacement. Feeling put upon, he decided to talk to a therapist. The therapist helped him refuse to adopt a victim mentality. "It's natural to ask, 'Why me?,'" counseled the therapist, "but this mentality doesn't help." Dirk continued to meet with the therapist as his medical journey continued.

In April 2019, Dirk underwent hip replacement surgery. After the procedure, while still at the hospital, a CT scan was performed to find the cause of a different issue—chronically numb feet. The neurologist called him the next day and told him his spine was collapsing and pinching the nerves to his feet. If not treated as soon as possible, it could leave him with a permanent drop foot; he would be unable to lift his foot when he walked. In consultation with the spine and the vascular surgeons, double spine surgery was scheduled.

So, four weeks later, in May 2019, and still walking with a cane from the hip replacement procedure, Dirk underwent his fifth surgery. During the subsequent ten days in the hospital, while having thoughts of *enough is enough*, he realized the support of his family had given him much to be thankful for. So once again he focused on healing.

As of this writing, Dirk is recovered and spends his time painting, reading, socializing with friends, and spending as much time with his family as possible.

LESSONS LEARNED

- An unexpected, life-threatening condition can trigger fear and panic. Dirk was able to rely on the comfort and support of his family to calm his emotional state.

- By developing rapport with his healthcare workers, Dirk was able to quiet the resistance and reduce his stress. He also learned to focus on his own healing by showing appreciation and gratitude to the people in his life.

- Recognizing the emotional trauma of repeated health issues, Dirk realized the need to seek professional help, which has contributed to his recovery and overall well-being.

WHAT YOU NEED TO KNOW

Dirk was fortunate to have survived multiple surgeries and hospitalizations. However, it is not uncommon, after so many recurring medical events, for a patient to experience a range of emotions, including fear, anxiety, anger, sadness, depression, or even some of the symptoms of PTSD (post-traumatic stress disorder) that have plagued veterans, who suffer from the trauma of war, and healthcare workers in a COVID-19 world. Patients can also suffer from ICU syndrome, with symptoms like fear, anxiety, depression, hallucinations, and delirium. In fact, family and friends can experience a form of ICU syndrome themselves because of the impact the time in the ICU had on their loved one and the subsequent behaviors following discharge.

Recognizing and naming these emotions is often the first step in dealing with them. While facing life-threatening medical procedures, Dirk was able to adopt a calm mental state that helped him through each crisis. He acknowledged and accepted his feelings and was not afraid to seek help from a mental health practitioner. He knew that asking for help is not a sign of weakness but a sign of strength.

While no single approach is right for everyone, there are several ways to help manage one's psychological and emotional health during a difficult time.

Family and Friends

Dirk was fortunate to have his wife's calming presence throughout his surgeries and convalescence. His sons brought joy and light into his life when he needed them most. On the ski vacation, he was lucky to have a physician friend to corroborate the diagnosis of the clinic's doctor and reassure him about the need for surgery at Grand Junction.

Unfortunately, not everyone has family or friends available to care for them and therefore must face circumstances like Dirk's alone. The COVID-19 pandemic has demonstrated unequivocally the importance of advocacy and human connection and the myriad negative impacts when they are not available. Sadly, patients stricken with the virus have had to be isolated from loved ones in the hospital, senior centers, and at home, and healthcare workers have labored diligently to provide needed support. This isolation during the pandemic has led to a three-to-four-fold increase in psychological and emotional distress. A *Journal of the American Medical Association* (*JAMA*) survey in September 2020 found U.S. adults were reporting levels of depressive symptoms more than three times higher during the pandemic than before it. And suffering in the mental health arena has extended beyond depression to include loneliness, anxiety, increased alcohol use, setbacks in addiction treatment, and suicide.[1]

Navigating the healthcare system, managing chronic medical conditions, and undergoing medical procedures can be a lonely experience. Research has shown that loneliness can have a deleterious effect on one's physical health equivalent to smoking fifteen cigarettes a day and can lead to serious mental health concerns.[2] Reaching out to others to talk, walk, or play can be an important way to stay mentally and emotionally healthy during these arduous times.

Therapies and Healing Methods

Below are options that may help an individual manage the psychological and emotional trauma of ongoing medical conditions. You may want to explore more than one approach or technique to find the one(s) most beneficial for your situation.

Talk therapy

You may benefit from therapy with a psychiatrist, psychologist, or other behavioral health professional. Finding the right trained professional who is a good fit for you is key to developing a trusting relationship and working together successfully. In Dirk's case, it proved helpful to talk through his negative thoughts and feelings. His therapist helped him gain perspective and positively manage his despondency. He discovered more fully the value and benefits of gratitude to one's health and well-being.

So, how do you find the individual who is the right fit? To find a therapist, you might want to start by asking your primary care practitioner for a recommendation. You can also talk to others, but remember: everyone's needs are unique. Students may have access to a university health or counseling center. Another resource is to check the website psychologytoday.com for a listing of licensed therapists in your city or zip code. A careful online search may also provide resources for various subgroups, such as communities of color and the LBGTQIA+ community. During the COVID pandemic, telehealth and virtual options made some mental health services more accessible.

Once you have the name of a therapist, call and talk for a few minutes. You should be able to quickly get a sense of whether the individual truly "hears" you, is nonjudgmental, and makes you feel comfortable. Don't be discouraged, however, if the therapist or healing practitioner is not the right fit for you. Many times, finding the right person is a trial-and-error process.

Cognitive behavioral therapy (CBT)

Cognitive behavioral therapy (CBT) is a structured treatment that focuses on negative thought patterns that have become automatic and reflexive but may not represent an objective view of one's situation. With the help of a trained therapist, one learns how to identify and reframe thoughts that negatively impact behaviors, emotions, and moods. CBT has been shown to be effective in addressing multiple conditions, including addiction, stress, anxiety, depression, and panic attacks. It is designed to provide coping skills that reduce the risk of negative, disturbing, or destructive thoughts that often lead to a black-and-white view of the world that is heavily weighted by pessimism and catastrophizing. CBT offers a more balanced perspective when assessing one's life circumstances.

Talking through one's feelings and emotions with a practitioner trained in CBT can be healing to the mind and the body. A therapist can help reveal the link between one's thoughts and emotions and one's physical and mental well-being.

Eye movement desensitization and reprocessing (EMDR)

Eye movement desensitization and reprocessing (EMDR) is a type of psychotherapy not based on talking or medication; it has a very structured protocol. By tracking a patient's eye movements when recalling a distressing event, the trained therapist can relieve the symptoms attached to that event. By forming new associations in the patient's mind, the therapist can unblock the traumatic event and promote mental healing.

Some conditions for which EMDR may be helpful include PTSD, sexual or other physical abuse, phobias, panic attacks, eating disorders, and grief.

Tapping

Tapping is a type of therapy that involves using your fingertips along certain points and channels (meridians) of the body while talking through distressing events and emotions to send signals to the brain. Studies indicate tapping, also known as the emotional freedom technique (EFT), is an evidence-based approach shown to be effective in addressing conditions such as anxiety, depression, phobias, and PTSD.

Zero balancing

Zero balancing is a technique that engages the body's energy to reduce stress and promote healing. Using gentle touch therapy at certain pressure points on the body (fully clothed), this treatment method can help release tension and promote relaxation and overall well-being.

Nature-based therapy (ecotherapy)

Research into nature-based therapy (ecotherapy) has shown that spending time in nature has a positive effect on physical and mental health and well-being. Actions as simple as viewing nature scenes can decrease muscle tension, reduce pain, and improve sleep. After spending time in the hospital and at home recuperating, being outdoors can be therapeutic. Walking by the ocean or in the woods can help relieve stress and restore a healthy immune system. A practice called *shinrin-yoku*, or "forest bathing," which originated in Japan, has become an increasingly popular form of ecotherapy.[3]

Animal therapy

Animals can help people cope with and recover from some physical and mental health conditions. Some hospitals have introduced service dogs to patients, particularly children. They produce a calming effect as they are petted and caressed. This soothing sensation can help reduce blood pressure, alleviate pain, and improve the patient's psychological state. At home, the unconditional loving companionship of a cat or dog can help reduce loneliness and anxiety and has been shown to improve overall cardiovascular health.

Equine-Assisted (Horse) Therapy has also been used to treat a variety of physical and emotional health issues and has been effective in adults, teens, and children. Horses are sensitive to emotions, and by feeding, grooming, leading, and riding a horse, children learn to bond and build a sense of trust with the horse. The interaction with a horse, along with a trained therapist, can provide a breakthrough when dealing with negative emotions and can promote healing.

Music/art/movement therapy

With a qualified therapist, past trauma can sometimes be healed through expressive therapies.

Music therapy—Music therapy has been shown to provide benefits in those with depression, anxiety, pain, and chronic illness. Certain songs can trigger memories and release pent-up emotions that talking cannot reach; they can enable one to change moods and emotions by changing music.

Art therapy—Art therapy is an integrative mental health treatment that uses applied psychological theory and the creative process of making art to address issues such as depression, anxiety, and PTSD. Art therapists are trained in both art and therapy. The creation of art can be used to express emotions, to develop coping skills that help ease emotional distress, and to gain insights and self-awareness to deal with life's challenges. You do not need any artistic ability to benefit from this form of therapy.

Dance/movement therapy—The American Dance Therapy Association (ADTA) defines dance therapy as "the psychotherapeutic use of movement to promote emotional, social, cognitive, and physical integration of the individual, for the purpose of improving health and well-being."[4]

Research has shown that movement therapy can lead to differences in brain structure and can be effective in those experiencing depression, Alzheimer's, and Parkinson's disease.

Moving your body to dance rhythms can be a therapeutic way to let go of tension, "exercise" the brain, improve balance and physical strength, and achieve human connection.

Neurofeedback

This is a type of biofeedback that uses an EEG (electroencephalogram) test to measure the electrical activity of the brain. A patient can see or receive a sound signal that demonstrates changes occurring with different thoughts and other stimuli. Knowing that our brains can continue to grow and change throughout our lives through neuroplasticity (how the brain forms new neural connections), we can learn to train ourselves to calm the electrical impulses in our brains and promote healing. Neurofeedback has been found to be helpful in a variety of conditions including stress and anxiety, PTSD, sleep disorders, and age-related cognitive loss.

Mindfulness, meditation, tai chi, and qigong

The following practices have been used for centuries to relieve emotional and physical distress and address health issues. The good news is that none of these take a lot of time or require equipment. Free videos can be found on the internet if you prefer a virtual experience or do not have access to an in-person class. As with doing any research on the internet, look for signs of legitimacy and individuals with the expertise to be leading a session.

Mindfulness—Jon Kabat-Zinn, often called the "father of mindfulness," and the founder of the Mindfulness-Based Stress Reduction (MBSR) program at the University of Massachusetts Medical Center, describes mindfulness as "awareness by paying attention in the present moment non-judgmentally as if it really mattered." It has been found to be effective in a variety of situations, including stress, chronic conditions like hypertension, and insomnia.

Mindfulness helps protect against stress and overwhelming feelings by building new neural pathways and can even change the relative size of certain parts of the brain. When engaging in negative self-talk, we can use mindfulness to aid in differentiating our thoughts and beliefs from objective facts and reality. Simply thinking something does not make it true.

Meditation—Although meditation and mindfulness are often used interchangeably; they can be similar but are not the same.[5] Meditation is one way to practice mindfulness, but there are others, like mindful eating. There are several ways to practice meditation to reduce stress and anxiety and become more emotionally calm.

Tai chi and qigong—These are ancient Chinese healing techniques that involve posture, movement, and deep breathing to treat a variety of health conditions. They have been used for centuries; the flow of energy through the body promotes healing and can bring overall well-being. These exercises have been used to improve mood and sleep, and to promote better balance and flexibility.

Practicing gratitude

Robert Emmons, a leading expert on gratitude, believes that two components make up gratitude: (1) an affirmation of goodness in the world and of the benefits we've received, and (2) the sources of this goodness are outside of ourselves.

Once we are the recipient of goodness, we gain a greater appreciation for what we have and a natural instinct to pay it forward. Benefits of a gratitude practice include greater mental and emotional well-being, as well as resilience, better sleep and heart health, fewer absences due to illness, greater job satisfaction, less cynicism, a greater sense of connection to others, and a reduced risk of depression and anxiety. Gratitude has also been shown to be effective in helping to address stress, suicide risk, and PTSD.

Spirituality

For many people going through serious medical conditions, religion and spirituality can play a large role in providing comfort, solace, hope, and faith in the possible. Prayers for healing, whether in formal houses of worship or alone at home, enable trust in a higher power to restore well-being.

There are many techniques and practices that are effective, both alone and in conjunction with medical therapy, to manage the emotional distress of health challenges and mental health disorders. Critical to relief and treatment are the acknowledgment of one's emotions, the willingness to search for resources that can help, and the perseverance to find those that will work best for you.

SO, WHAT CAN YOU DO NOW?

- Your emotional health is inextricably intertwined with your physical health. To achieve optimal well-being, you need to take care of both. Do not hesitate to seek help. To recognize your emotional health needs and address them is a sign of strength, not a sign of weakness.

- Invest the time to explore your options and resources to determine the best fit for you.

- Recognize that your emotional health may change over time, and you may want to try a new method, or resume a prior one, depending on your situation.

- Focus on being present and grateful to help give you the resilience to get through the inevitable ups and downs of your health and well-being throughout life.

CHAPTER 9

Dealing with Mental Illness

I wish people could understand that the brain is the most important organ of our body. Just because you can't see mental illness like you could see a broken bone, doesn't mean it's not as detrimental or devastating to a family or an individual.

DEMI LOVATO

LINDA'S STORY ABOUT ELLEN

Linda's daughter Ellen began to display temper tantrums at about the age of seven. Although she had good grades in school, Ellen had difficulty making friends and getting along with others. In seventh grade, Ellen began seeing a therapist, but the difficulties continued. By the time she was ready to attend high school, Ellen refused to go to the nearby high school in her district and insisted on attending a different one, using the excuse of wanting to study Chinese. Her refusal more likely stemmed from anticipated difficulty with relationships at the assigned school.

While at home on a break from her first year of college, Ellen borrowed the family car, telling her parents she was looking for a summer job. Instead, she drove herself to the nearby hospital, informing the staff she was hearing voices and was afraid she was going to hurt the family dog. The hospital was not equipped to handle mental health patients, so they called Linda to pick up Ellen and take her to the larger regional hospital that had a psychiatric unit.

At the larger hospital, Ellen was admitted to the adult wing, where the other patients were much older, mostly in their fifties and sixties. There were no other young adults present. Ellen was given Haldol, a first-generation antipsychotic drug used to treat schizophrenia. Haldol can have potentially severe side effects, including tardive dyskinesia (involuntary movements of the face, trunk, and extremities), neuroleptic malignant syndrome (a rare reaction to antipsychotic drugs resulting in fever, muscle stiffness, sweating, unstable blood pressure, autonomic dysfunction, and stupor). Throughout her two-week stay at the hospital, Ellen remained heavily drugged and, according to Linda, in a zombie-like state.

Linda was very worried about her daughter. Ellen didn't belong there, she thought, and the treatment was not helping. Linda began to research other facilities. She learned about the Community Mental Health Act of 1963, signed by President John F. Kennedy, which provided federal funding for community centers specifically for the care of people with mental illnesses. Linda continued her research, contacting a range of people she knew, and discovered the local county's Community Services Board (CSB), a part of Virginia's state mental health plan. The CSB suggested that Ellen be transferred to a smaller private psychiatric hospital with a specific unit for young adults. The facility also had different levels of care, which meant patients did not have to be confined to a single room and could enjoy some additional privileges, depending on their condition. Ellen was assigned a psychiatrist to treat a diagnosis of schizophrenia, and she stayed for one month.

After Ellen's discharge, Linda wondered what to do next. Ellen could not be left alone, but living at home with her parents was too difficult. Linda and her husband both had full-time jobs. Ellen dropped out of college, slept most of the day, and took the car to go out. At times, Ellen even slept in the car. Given her condition, Ellen returned to the hospital's young adult section, received inpatient therapy, and continued to see the same psychiatrist. In preparation for discharge, an aftercare plan was developed, with attention to daily activities and future goals.

Linda learned there was a mental health center in the community that offered a daycare program that included group counseling and some limited art and music therapy. She enrolled her daughter, and Ellen continued to see the same psychiatrist on a weekly basis. However, the daycare program wasn't enough. Ellen needed to learn some life skills. Where would she live? Could she hold a job? Would she be able to manage her money and support herself? Would she be able to return to college?

Further research led Linda to another community organization that provided psychiatric rehabilitation services to individuals and their families. Using specialized counselors, they offered a recovery program to help adults with mental illness find and keep jobs, develop social skills, manage finances and nutrition, and maintain housing.

Knowing that Ellen could not live at home, Linda used her networking skills to find a nonprofit, charitable organization in her community that provided non-time-limited housing and supportive services to adults with serious mental illness. They placed Ellen in a group townhouse with three other women. The house had a counselor who came several hours per week to supervise and support the residents. Ellen learned to get along with her housemates and share the responsibilities of the house.

Ellen continued to maintain her relationship with the same psychiatrist for the next fifteen years. Because of the continued medication, Ellen was required to have periodic blood tests to detect any potential effects on her liver. Ellen used the family car for these appointments and other transportation needs.

As she grew older, Ellen never went back to college but worked a series of jobs, including in a fast-food restaurant, a bakery, a drugstore, and a retail clothing store.

Today, Ellen is fifty-two years old. She lives in a one-bedroom condo, as the group townhouse roommate mix became psychiatrically complicated over time. Ellen is not able to work but receives Social Security Disability Insurance (SSDI) benefits. No longer driving, she has learned to use public transportation, and her parents provide additional rides as needed.

Ellen's parents see her regularly and help take her to appointments. They set up a special needs trust for Ellen and designated their son as the executor. With the help of a few other close relatives, Ellen's brother will look after her when her parents are gone.

LESSONS LEARNED

- Mental illness carries a stigma in our society and can be very destructive for individuals and their families. Dealing with mental health conditions can be confusing, isolating, and dangerous. There may be challenges getting care due to an insufficient number of clinicians, inpatient beds, and available outpatient programs. Depending on an individual's age and the complexity of the condition, finding the appropriate resources can be even more difficult and takes perseverance.

- In addition to receiving the right treatment, individuals with serious mental illness may also need help with everyday life issues—housing and transportation needs, finding and keeping a job, and building and maintaining relationships in a culture that often fears and shuns people with behavioral health conditions—that usually don't exist for physical health challenges. It can put a tremendous burden on both the patient and the family to avoid falling into homelessness or becoming a victim of violence.

- Ellen was fortunate her mother was such a strong advocate for her. Linda was incredibly resourceful and discovered several organizations that existed right in her backyard.

WHAT YOU NEED TO KNOW

According to the National Alliance on Mental Illness (NAMI), one in every five adults in the United States will experience some mental illness each year.[1] One in twenty U.S. adults will experience a serious mental illness. As a result of the recent coronavirus pandemic, the number of adults and children experiencing anxiety and depression has skyrocketed.

Moreover, experts are saying the added stress and psychological trauma of isolation and feelings of loss have created additional stress and psychological trauma that may have long-term effects. Healthcare workers and first responders continue to suffer from PTSD in record numbers.

Diagnosing a mental health illness can be complicated, because there may not be a definitive test for all types of conditions. Additionally, while we may feel comfortable talking about physical illnesses, like cancer or diabetes, mental health issues can be difficult to speak about openly. Many people are still reluctant to share their condition, fear reprisal, and keep their problems hidden. Others may not know how best to respond, may avoid the individual, or may simply attribute a person's behavior to being "odd."

Some Mental Health Conditions

There are a number of mental health conditions that can vary in severity from one person to another and manifest themselves in different ways. Some symptoms may appear in childhood or adolescence, and others may surface later in life. There may be no one cause for these conditions; rather, the illness may be due to a variety of reasons, such as genetics, trauma, environment, lifestyle, stress, or chemical processes in the brain. They often require a combination of treatment options—including therapy and medication—to be managed successfully.

Unfortunately, many people suffer alone and become estranged from their families and friends. Those with severe symptoms may be unable to hold a traditional job to support themselves, become homeless, and, tragically, die or commit suicide. Additionally, for some, the side effects of the medications to treat the condition may be perceived as worse than the condition itself, causing some to stop taking their meds. For others, once the medication kicks in and resolves the symptoms, they may feel their life is under control and think the meds are no longer needed. Both situations can result in volatility in treatment and a cycle of symptom remissions and flares. Having support and encouragement to maintain adherence is critical to optimize the best outcomes. It is key to seek help early and often and persist in obtaining the right level of assistance to manage the condition effectively and live the most productive life possible.

Anxiety

Some level of apprehension is expected when giving a presentation to a large group or going for a job interview, for example. However, people with anxiety worry excessively and may suffer from panic attacks, situations in which their heart pounds and races, along with a shortness of breath and even chest pain that can feel like a heart attack. Fears and phobias often become overwhelming and can result in major challenges to daily functioning.

Attention deficit hyperactivity disorder (ADHD)

Attention deficit hyperactivity disorder (ADHD) is characterized by hyperactivity, difficulty paying attention, and challenges with impulse control. It is typically diagnosed during childhood, although, in some cases, it may not be officially recognized until adulthood. ADHD may negatively impact learning, organizational ability, and performance in school or at work, as well as relationships with others. There may be specific, state-mandated school programs and resources available to children with ADHD, so it is important to research the support that may exist in your community. However, be on the alert for inaccurate labeling and potentially unnecessary treatment with drugs in children who are simply fidgety with pent-up energy or boredom, due to lack of physical exercise perhaps, or for failure to recognize an exceptionally gifted student who has the talent to be placed at a higher grade level.

Bipolar disorder

People with bipolar disorder experience extreme shifts in moods—very high or manic behavior, followed by very low or depressive behavior—that can be unpredictable and uncontrollable. In a manic state, individuals may become irritable, irrational, or delusional and experience racing thoughts and pressured speech. They may engage in behaviors like excessive shopping far beyond need and the ability to pay, sexual promiscuity, and gambling. When in a depressive state, there may be a swing to feelings of hopelessness and perhaps a struggle to get out of bed. There are two categories of bipolar disorder, bipolar 1 and bipolar 2. Individuals with bipolar 2 have less severe manic episodes.

Borderline personality disorder (BPD)

In borderline personality disorder (BPD), individuals usually have an intense fear of abandonment or instability. This condition is characterized by wide mood swings, an inability to regulate emotions, extreme anger, a poor self-image, and impulsive or risky behavior. Lacking the tolerance for being alone, they often have intense, unstable relationships. Ironically and tragically, the very behaviors that result from BPD often drive others away, further exacerbating the fear of being abandoned.

Dementia

Dementia refers to a decline in the functioning of the brain in memory, reasoning, and other thinking skills. Alzheimer's disease is the most common type of dementia, followed by dementia due to cerebrovascular disease, like stroke. As the disease progresses, individuals can become disoriented and confused. Eventually they may be unable to function at all and become bedbound. While it is often associated with old age, dementia is not inevitable. As more research is done, we are learning more about possible lifestyle behaviors that may contribute to the disease and actions that can be taken to reduce risk, such as those described in Chapter 2. A search for an effective treatment to slow progression, as well as a cure to prevent or reverse the brain's decline, continues.

Depression

While we all may have feelings of sadness and disappointment at certain times in our lives, individuals with depression have persistent negative thoughts and experience prolonged periods of hopelessness, sometimes lasting months or even years. According to NAMI (National Alliance on Mental Illness), depression is a leading cause of disability worldwide.[2] People with depression have a higher risk of developing cardiovascular and metabolic disease. And those with chronic conditions like heart disease and diabetes are more likely to become depressed.

Eating disorders

People with eating disorders have an obsession and preoccupation with food and their body weight. Left untreated, these conditions can lead to severe illness and death. Eating disorders are most common among teen girls and young women in their twenties, when appearance and body image can be a primary focus. However, rising rates of eating disorders are being recognized in boys and men, accounting for up to 30 percent of the conditions.[3] Often, these self-destructive behaviors are kept hidden from family members and are not noticed until visible health problems arise.

- People with anorexia restrict their intake of food, thereby limiting the nutrition needed for their bodies to function. They can become noticeably thin—even emaciated—and their bodily functions begin to shut down.

- People who suffer from bulimia binge on large quantities of food and then purge their bodies through vomiting, laxatives, or other means, as a pattern of behavior to avoid the weight gain that would result from food bingeing. Over time, these continual vomiting episodes can result in dehydration, damage to the teeth and the digestive system, and cardiac problems. Some individuals will continue to binge large amounts of food in a short amount of time, well past the point of no longer being hungry. They often struggle with self-image and self-control.

- Those with eating disorders may also experience body dysmorphic disorder, which is a distinctly different condition characterized by extreme concern about outward appearance and a debilitating perception of body flaws that may be unnoticeable to others or not exist at all.

Obsessive compulsive disorder (OCD)

People with obsessive compulsive disorder (OCD) may suffer from obsessions and/or compulsions. They can exhibit uncontrollable, repetitive behaviors resulting from irrational thoughts and fears, such as repeatedly turning off the stove, locking a door, or washing one's hands. Sometimes the behavior is self-destructive, such as pulling out one's hair from eyebrows, eyelashes, or the head. Hoarding is another manifestation of OCD that can severely impact living conditions, including potential threats to safety and hygiene.

Post-traumatic stress disorder (PTSD)

Traumatic or extremely stressful events can have an impact on one's mental health, as seen with war veterans, 9/11 survivors, those with long ICU stays, healthcare workers caring for COVID-19 patients, and, as mentioned in Chapter 8, people who have experienced severe medical conditions. PTSD sufferers may become agitated or fearful, may ruminate over triggering events, and sometimes experience flashbacks and hallucinations. They may also experience anxiety and/or depression related to their PTSD.

Schizophrenia

Schizophrenia is a complex mental illness that affected 3.2 million in the U.S. in 2021,[4] with the typical onset in males in the late teens and women in their twenties and thirties. Symptoms may include hallucinations—such as hearing voices—delusions, and mental confusion. It may first surface with a psychotic break—a sudden onset of irrational behavior, delusions, or hallucinations—and requires professional help. Untreated, it can be quite challenging to get or keep a job, interact with others, and achieve a stable life. Contrary to popular misconceptions, most who suffer from schizophrenia do not pose a threat to others and are not violent. Unfortunately, it is not uncommon for many with schizophrenia to end up homeless or incarcerated. Fortunately, over time, more effective medications have been developed to treat the condition, as well as reduce the likelihood of commonly seen side effects.

Substance use disorder

Continued, impulsive use of alcohol or drugs despite negative consequences remains a serious problem in the U.S. As a result of the opioid crisis, as well as the pandemic, addiction to drugs and alcohol has been on the rise. According to the CDC, the accidental drug overdose rate exceeded 100,000 in 2021, an increase of 28.5 percent.[5] New treatments, focused on preventing self-harm and/or managing the addiction, have increased. Peer groups for individuals—as well as family members—including AA (Alcoholics Anonymous), Al-Anon, and Narcotics Anonymous, are often effective forms of ongoing support.

With the proper treatment, most of these conditions can be managed so individuals can lead stable, productive lives. It is important to remember there's no shame in being diagnosed with a mental health condition or in seeking the help you need. Like physical health conditions, you and/or your family benefit by being proactive when signs and symptoms appear, recur, or flare. Your mental health is as important as your physical well-being, and the two are inextricably intertwined.

Signs and Symptoms

We all feel down or anxious at times, but how do you know if you're experiencing something more serious, or even life threatening? Is it just a matter of degree, severity, frequency, or the length of time symptoms persist? According to NAMI, the following are common signs in adults and adolescents that may signal a mental health challenge or condition for which professional help is often needed:

- Excessive worrying or fear
- Feeling excessively sad or low
- Confused thinking or problems concentrating and learning
- Extreme mood changes, including uncontrollable "highs" or feelings of euphoria
- Prolonged or strong feelings of irritability or anger
- Avoiding friends and social activities
- Difficulties understanding or relating to other people
- Changes in sleeping habits or feeling tired and low energy
- Changes in eating habits, such as increased hunger or lack of appetite
- Changes in sex drive
- Delusions or hallucinations, for example, hearing voices or seeing things that don't exist in objective reality
- Inability to perceive changes in one's own feelings, behavior, or personality, or being unaware of one's own mental health condition (anosognosia)
- Overuse of substances like alcohol or drugs
- Multiple physical ailments without obvious causes (such as headaches, stomach aches, vague and ongoing aches and pains)
- Thoughts about suicide
- Inability to carry out daily activities or handle daily problems and stress
- An intense fear of weight gain or concern with appearance, cycles of gorging or bingeing followed by self-induced vomiting

According to the National Institute for Health Care Management (NIHCM) Foundation,[6] 75 percent of mental health disorders develop by age twenty-four. Prior to the pandemic, one child out of five was diagnosed with a mental health condition. Since the onset of the pandemic—with school closures, social isolation, economic instability, and loss of a family member—emotional distress in children has surged, and rates of depression have increased. Suicide is reported as the second leading cause of death among children.

In young children and adolescents, it often can be difficult to determine whether certain behaviors are normal and temporary or may be signs of deeper mental health issues. These include:

- Changes in school performance
- Excessive worry or anxiety, for example, fighting to avoid bed or school
- Hyperactive behavior
- Frequent nightmares
- Frequent disobedience or aggression
- Frequent temper tantrums

Where to Go for Information

In every U.S. state, the Department of Human Services has a division of mental health. In most states, the mental health unit is called the Division of Mental Health and Addiction Services (DMHAS). Under the agency, you can find information about the national Substance Abuse and Mental Health Services Administration (SAMHSA).

Under federal law, the agency oversees community-based behavioral services, such as:

- Substance abuse prevention and early intervention
- Emergency screening
- Intensive outpatient mental health services
- Addiction services, partial care, and partial hospitalization
- Case management
- Medication-assisted treatment for substance abuse

In some states, funds may be available for individuals of low socioeconomic status in need of short- and long-term mental health and substance abuse residential services. Additionally, the nationally known Program of Assertive Community Treatment (PACT) may offer some residential programs. PACT is an evidence-based intervention that helps those with mental health conditions as they transition back to the community. The program provides support for employment, education, and housing.

Guardianship

If a patient with mental illness is declared incompetent, a family member may be granted guardianship and have access to the patient's medical records. A surrogate's court may allow guardianship over an intellectually or developmentally disabled individual (depending on the degree of disability), such as those with Down syndrome, cerebral palsy, or autism. Guardianship may also be granted for an individual who cannot take care of him or herself due to old age, Alzheimer's and other dementias, or traumatic brain injury (TBI).

Tragically, in cases of children with ongoing severe mental illness who are insufficiently responsive to treatment and present a threat to their own safety and/or that of their families, it may not be possible for them to remain in the home.

Given the current limitations of mental health services and a cost that may be out of reach, it is sometimes the case that families end up relinquishing custody to the state so their loved one can obtain the level of care that's needed.

The pandemic has caused an increase in the emotional distress and mental health of both adults and children. Though some have suffered much more grief and loss, everyone has felt at least some degree of stress, trauma, or angst. As a result, we have seen a big step forward in the increased awareness of mental health and the importance of seeking help.

However, there is no one solution to addressing the needs of those with mental health conditions, as each person's history, symptoms, and family dynamics may be different. Just like physical illnesses, it's important to seek healthcare professionals who take your symptoms and concerns seriously and treat you with respect. Empowering yourself to take charge of your mental well-being is just as important as the actions you take about your physical health.

SO, WHAT CAN YOU DO NOW?

- You are not alone. Mental health issues are common and have been exacerbated by the COVID-19 pandemic. Acknowledge the problem. Admitting there is a problem is the first step. If the condition is impacting your normal functioning—your work, family, friends, physical health—then it's time to seek help.

- Don't keep your problems hidden, and don't ignore the warning signs and symptoms. Avoid feeling shame or blaming yourself.

- Reach out. Share your feelings with a trusted friend or family member who won't criticize or shame you and can provide support.

- Communicate with your healthcare practitioner if you are concerned about yourself or a loved one. It is not unusual for mental health issues to be associated with physical medical conditions. If you have an open and honest relationship with your physician, you should be able to talk about your anxieties, fears, addictions, and other behavioral problems. Medical ethics and laws like HIPAA mean the doctor may not share this information without your permission. And mental health conditions tend to fall in a category with an additional level of protection relative to privacy and confidentiality. Your physician may not be experienced in treating a mental health condition but can refer you to a specialist who is.

- Learn more. Just like any physical illness, it is equally important to educate yourself about the condition. Put a name to it if you can and see if the symptoms match yours.

- Explore the various treatment options. As discussed in Chapter 8, a variety of therapies exist to treat mental health issues. Medication is not always necessary, but when it is, it might be combined with other treatment modalities. If a condition becomes severe enough (or even life threatening), an inpatient stay or residential facility may be appropriate to provide round-the-clock care.

- Investigate any local resources that may be available in your community, including therapists, support groups, and specific health facilities. Find out if there are medical professionals or facilities that specialize in treating your condition. Just as Ellen's mother discovered, there may be resources in your area that offer treatment and support recovery. Individual and group facilities may provide access to affordable therapy, housing, and work support.

- Check your health insurance plan. As with physical ailments, you will want to see what limitations exist (e.g., number of therapy sessions, dollar limit, etc.).

- If you or a loved one is in crisis, seek help immediately. Call a help line and/or go to a nearby health facility. As of July 16, 2022, the number **988** was designated as the first-ever three-digit dialing and text code for suicide prevention and mental health crisis. Calls are routed to the nearest call center (over two hundred in the U.S.) or the national backup network.

CHAPTER 10

Facing Health Disparities

Eliminating disparities requires truly patient-centered care—that is, individualized care by clinicians who appreciate that patients' beliefs, behaviors, social and economic challenges, and environments dictate their health outcomes.

MARSHALL CHIN, MD

CAROL'S STORY

Carol grew up in a small town in Indiana, about five miles from Louisville, Kentucky. The town was predominantly white, with a small Black population and no Black doctors.

Carol lived with her mother and stepfather; she didn't meet her biological father until much later in life. The family was extremely poor and could not afford health insurance. As a child, Carol never saw a physician except for the accidental injuries from her "tomboy" adventures. There was no money for dental visits either.

As Carol reached puberty and began to menstruate, her periods became increasingly painful, and even more so by the time she reached her late teens and early twenties. Sometimes the pain was so excruciating she could barely eat, afraid to create any additional pressure in her abdomen. Her mother was "old school," and never sought medical help. With little formal education herself, her mother never openly talked to her about sex or reproduction.

After high school, Carol enrolled at the local community college to study computer science, but she also needed to work to support herself. Taking classes while holding a full-time job became too difficult, and she dropped out to devote her energies to earning a much-needed income.

At age twenty-seven, Carol's menstrual cycle got worse; the bleeding wouldn't stop. She had never been to a gynecologist before, so her mother took Carol to the emergency room. Her blood count had become so low that she was diagnosed with anemia. The ER staff couldn't believe that Carol was able to walk into the hospital without assistance.

A gynecologist was assigned at the hospital. After the examination, Carol was told she needed a D&C (dilation and curettage), a procedure to remove tissue from inside the uterus to diagnose and treat the heavy bleeding. But Carol had just started a new job, and her health insurance coverage had not yet kicked in.

Carol needed the procedure desperately, but knew she couldn't afford the hospital bill. However, not wanting to withhold the needed procedure, the hospital offered to help. The billing office representative said if Carol could take time off from her new job for one month, the county would pay the bill. Fortunately, Carol was able to take the time off, the bill was paid, and her new employer collected donations to help Carol meet some of her financial obligations. Carol was extremely grateful, given that she hadn't even been at her new job one month and didn't know anyone yet.

Weeks later, Carol returned to work and finally was able to obtain health insurance after ninety days. The gynecologist put her on birth control pills to control the bleeding, as the D&C did not help. Carol didn't like the way the birth control pills made her feel, and she often became nauseated.

"There's a new experimental injection I can give you," said the gynecologist. "It costs five hundred dollars a month, however." There was no way Carol could afford it, and she didn't know to explore whether her new insurance would pay for any experimental treatment. She also had a phobia about injections from her experiences as a child getting stitches after her accidental injuries.

So, with her ongoing painful periods and continued bleeding, the doctor informed her—falsely—that the only other option was to have a hysterectomy. The doctor appeared barely older than Carol. At age twenty-seven, Carol didn't fully understand the implications of having a hysterectomy. She did realize this meant she would never be able to have children but didn't know the surgery could result in the abrupt onset of menopause, with many of the associated and sometimes debilitating symptoms some women experience, such as night sweats, fatigue, and brain fog, as well as the earlier onset of increased risks of conditions like heart disease and osteoporosis.

Carol wasn't told and didn't know there were other options to treat the fibroids that were causing the bleeding. She didn't know that fibroids are growths that can develop in or on a woman's uterus or that they are usually non-cancerous but can become quite large and cause severe abdominal pain and heavy periods. She also did not know they are much more common in Black women. In 1986, the technology to freeze a woman's eggs was available, but Carol wasn't offered that option, which would have allowed another woman to carry a child for her in the future through surrogacy. With no money, little knowledge, and lacking a family advocate, Carol had nowhere else to turn.

So, in the spring of 1989, at age twenty-seven, Carol underwent a partial hysterectomy, removing her uterus but leaving the ovaries. She was not given the option of having a less invasive, laparoscopic hysterectomy, and an abdominal hysterectomy was done instead. She left the hospital with no understanding of what to expect after the surgery or how her body could change because of the procedure. With this life-altering surgery at such a young age, Carol did not realize, at the time, the psychological implications of never being able to have her own biological children.

Carol spent the next six weeks off work recovering from the surgery. She liked to sew and spent much of the time buying fabric to create a new wardrobe of clothes for her eventual return to work. She was determined to focus on her career.

In 2007, Carol needed a breast reduction to decrease the size of her breasts. After getting a second opinion, she decided to move forward with the second surgeon, as the first surgeon indicated she would have "bat wings" under her arms if she performed the surgery. Carol had the surgery and was very pleased at losing eight pounds related to the breast tissue that was removed. She had relatives who helped her with the drains and bandages.

Postoperatively, the surgeon informed Carol not to lift her arms any higher than putting a plate in a microwave, and she did as she was instructed. Unfortunately, the surgeon failed to tell her that, after a certain period of time, she should begin to move her arms in circular motions. As a result, she ended up with frozen shoulder syndrome, unable to even hook or unhook her bra "or wipe her own backside properly" and had to start physical therapy to get a partial range of motion back. She continued to have difficulty lifting her arms. Carol feels she should have given feedback to the surgeon, but she was transitioning to another big career change within the next six months.

In 2010, Carol began having more severe night sweats and other menopause symptoms. She found a new gynecologist, who started her on an HRT (hormone replacement therapy) regimen for a year, including estrogen patches and creams. No one informed Carol about any potential side effects or risks.

In 2011, Carol went to her gynecologist and said, "I am having a problem getting to the bathroom in time." She had become incontinent and was referred to a urogynecologist, a specialist with expertise in issues related to a woman's pelvic floor, like uterine prolapse and urinary incontinence. After a series of imaging studies, the urogynecologist identified a growth that was wrapped around her colon and resting on top of her bladder. *This is why I'm having problems with incontinence*, she thought.

Carol's gynecologist referred her to an oncologist to remove the growth, but that doctor was not available for some time. So, Carol turned to a cousin who knew another gynecologist specializing in cancer surgery.

Using the latest robotic technology, the growth was removed along with the rest of her female reproductive organs. Carol was relieved the problem was treated, but now reminded she could never have a child, her sinking sadness returned. She continued estrogen therapy and thought the incontinence problem was resolved.

But Carol's problems continued. A routine mammogram in November 2013 revealed a potential problem in her left breast. An appointment was scheduled for additional imaging at the local hospital, with a biopsy to be performed the day after Thanksgiving. It was cancer. She would have to start a chemotherapy regimen as soon as possible.

"What do I do now?" Carol worried. "I am about to start a different job. Should I stay with my old job now or go forward with the new one?"

She decided to speak to the human resources (HR) representative during her first week of new employment. "I don't want my manager to know about my cancer," Carol told HR. Carol was concerned her employer might believe going through chemo would mean she could not perform her new job. Carol obtained health insurance after the thirty-day waiting period. She couldn't afford to take a medical leave of absence without pay (FMLA) but was allowed to work a modified schedule so she could receive a chemo treatment each week.

And so, beginning in January 2014, Carol began receiving chemotherapy injections after having a port surgically implanted in her upper right chest area. Each treatment was very painful. The oncology center gave her some cream to apply to the port area and covered it with plastic wrap for thirty minutes to numb the area prior to the injections. However, the numbing cream didn't help, and Carol would take a deep breath with every sharp pain of the needle. She subsequently lost all her hair and received a free wig from the American Cancer Society. She bought other wigs as well.

For the next six months, Carol worked a four-day week and received her chemo treatment every Thursday. Because she had no vacation time and would have been unable to survive on FMLA with no pay, the six months were a terrible ordeal. She was given steroids to reduce the effects of the chemo, but they made her feel hyped up and edgy. Carol developed a blood clot behind her chemo port and had to do the thing she hated most—give herself a daily abdominal shot to help dissolve the clot. The shot "burned like fire." It was a vicious cycle to go to work, come home, undergo the chemo treatment each week, and never feel rested from the drugs and steroids. Yet, despite her exhaustion, Carol steadily managed to attend church for support.

During this time, Carol met with the cancer surgeon, who thought the estrogen therapy could be the likely cause of her breast cancer. She stopped the estrogen patch and creams immediately. Carol discovered later that this specific estrogen therapy was correlated with her exact type of breast cancer.

One day, while Carol was at church, she spoke with a woman who was known to have a healing gift. The woman put her hand on Carol's head and began to pray for her. Carol immediately collapsed in the pew and sobbed.

Prior to the completion of the six-month chemo regimen, Carol believed she was healed and was getting better. "I think I am healed," Carol told the oncology team. Carol asked to be tested with additional imaging to see if the cancer was gone. "Well, if we do images now, and you still have cancer, the insurance won't pay for more imaging at the time of surgery," the oncology team representative responded.

Upset that the person refused to believe her and uncomfortable with the environment at the cancer center, she pursued a second opinion from another oncologist at a different cancer center that a previous coworker had used. The new physician listened as Carol explained the previous diagnosis. He examined her and said, "If I had known you for the past ten to thirteen years, I wouldn't believe you had cancer."

The new physician called the first surgeon, who said Carol was mistaken regarding the extent of the cancer and its prognosis. However, Carol knew the cancer surgeon had shown her the breast x-ray with the cancer present. The surgeon had discussed the treatment plan, that both breasts would need to be removed and then reconstructed, and even discussed the name of a good plastic surgeon. In addition, Carol's primary care physician at the time called her to discuss the cancer prognosis, affirmed that she needed both breasts removed, and mentioned that a niece had the same type of cancer.

After chemo was completed, surgery was scheduled. Carol chose to stay with the first surgeon despite the controversy. Carol insisted she was healed and instructed her surgeon to check first to see if the cancer was still there. On the day of her surgery, the surgeon said, "I'm going to do what you want, Carol." (Carol learned later her surgeon didn't sleep all night before her surgery, worried that Carol was making the wrong decision for her body.)

The surgeon, in accordance with Carol's wishes, removed two or three lymph nodes and had them tested. The markers that had been placed in the breast where the cancer had been present were removed, a small lumpectomy was performed to examine part of the breast tissue where the cancer was previously seen, and the cancer port was surgically removed, too.

Remarkably, there was no cancer! Was this the result of the chemo? Or was this the result of prayer and the hand of God? Carol believes it was the latter. She had stage 3 breast cancer, and now it was gone—no cancer could be found!

Carol was informed by the surgeon that she would always have fragments of the cancer in her breast if they weren't removed and that every year Carol would be wondering if she truly had cancer or just calcifications. From then on, Carol scheduled her mammograms every year, and each time there were no calcifications and no further presence of cancer. Years later, Carol discovered that her medical record indicated the lumpectomy biopsy but failed to reflect the healing of her cancer after the chemo.

Carol praises Jesus when she thinks about how he healed her. She often cries, when taking a shower, wondering how women live without their natural breasts and the sorrow they must feel.

After reading more about the estrogen treatment, Carol returned to have a discussion with the gynecologist who prescribed the hormone replacement therapy. "You need to inform women about the risks of this treatment," she told the doctor. "I had an intraductal carcinoma caused by this estrogen therapy, and I don't want other women to go through what I did." The doctor responded that other women had been prescribed the same HRT, and they were fine.

As of this writing, Carol continues to follow up with her oncologist twice a year and remains cancer-free. However, because of the chemo, she experiences some ongoing neuropathy (dysfunction of one or more peripheral nerves, typically causing numbness, weakness, or coldness) in her hands and feet. She also has been under the care of an eye doctor after experiencing some strange "spirals" in her eyes during the chemo treatment period. The eye doctor is watching her closely for the potential development of glaucoma.

In addition, Carol's heart was affected. In 2019, after the discovery that her heart's ability to pump blood had diminished to 40 percent, Carol had to undergo cardiac rehab therapy for nine months and is still being monitored by a cardiologist. She lost confidence in her cardiologist based on some failed treatment and now has a new one, referred by her primary care physician, to manage her care.

About to turn sixty, Carol experienced severe incontinence due to problems with her pelvic floor and saw another specialist for the condition. Despite a long waiting period to get an appointment, Carol was able to see the doctor, who confirmed that she did have a weak pelvic floor. The doctor prescribed some medicine for two months to get the incontinence under control and advised her to see a physical therapist who could teach Carol how to properly do Kegel exercises to strengthen her pelvic floor. Carol independently researched the value of Kegel exercises and was frustrated no healthcare provider ever informed her about this technique since her original surgery in 1989. No one counseled her about menopause or keeping her weight down when she was only slightly overweight back then. And no one ever suggested or provided any mental health counseling to help with the continuing despair of not being able to have children and its impact on her emotional well-being as she got older.

Today, after so many healthcare system failures and often not receiving information regarding potential options and side effects, Carol feels the healthcare system and many of her doctors let her down. She regrets not having the ability to have children and would like to be married. "Who would want to marry a woman who has so many health problems?" she lamented. "No one told me what to expect or explained my options. I didn't know enough even to ask questions. We were so poor, and as a Black female, I think I was just written off."

To take charge of her health now, she has sought counseling through the help of the EAP (Employee Assistance Program) benefit from her employer. To reduce weight, she watches her eating habits and has joined a gym to participate in a strength training class. She bought a Fitbit fitness tracker to monitor her activity and has a health coach for support. She had her heart tested again, and her blood flow has now increased from 40 percent to 45 percent.

Since her mother and stepfather have passed, she has formed a close relationship with her aunt and talks to her every day. Carol did participate in raising some young relatives but didn't feel a mother-child connection in the relationship. She was glad, however, to have helped some children in her life.

LESSONS LEARNED

- The healthcare system, like life itself, can be unfair and inequitable. Certain segments of the population—including women, communities of color, those with a lower economic status, and those living in a rural area—are more likely to experience health disparities and provider bias. In her younger years, many of these factors applied to Carol. Unfortunately, she experienced a scarcity of healthcare services, and the dismissiveness of her healthcare practitioners contributed to a series of avoidable consequences—physical, mental, and emotional.

- Carol became a victim of a system of healthcare practitioners who provided limited information about her medical conditions and treatment options and failed to explain the long-term implications of their procedures. Her frustration and depression grew to a distrust of the doctors and of the healthcare system itself.

- She learned how important it is to be knowledgeable about one's body and any health issues that one may experience. Armed with a baseline understanding of her medical conditions, she learned the importance of asking questions, gathering information about all treatment options, discussing the pros and cons, and making the best decision for oneself.

- In the end, Carol found her power, learned to advocate for herself, and took charge of her health and well-being.

WHAT YOU NEED TO KNOW

Carol's story demonstrates the complexity of the healthcare system and the critical need for a focus on the patient as a whole person—body, mind, and spirit—in collaboration with a culturally competent medical practitioner. As with all patients, Carol needed a healthcare provider who would ensure she understood her condition without dismissing or ignoring her concerns, made the time to discuss all available options, and shared decision-making while taking her health beliefs and preferences into account. All too often, patients bear the burden of the inherent power imbalance between patient and doctor, highlighting the need for training in medical school (and other professional healthcare programs) beyond just teaching about disease. At some of the most vulnerable and frightening times of their lives, patients are expected to understand a serious condition with unfamiliar terminology and make decisions with often unknown consequences and frequently in a short amount of time. And patients must do all this without the critical advocacy skills needed to effectively navigate the healthcare system and obtain the affordable, high-quality, cost-effective care they want and deserve.

Thankfully, Carol had the strength and resilience to overcome myriad challenges. She is now taking action to help reduce the likelihood that others will have similar experiences. However, not everyone is able to overcome long-standing racial and ethnic biases and the many health disparities that patients face.

By definition, health disparities are health differences related to social, economic, and/or environmental disadvantages that adversely affect people based on factors such as race, ethnicity, sex, gender identity, age, socioeconomic status, geographic location, or disability. The National Institutes of Health defines health disparities as "the difference in the incidence, prevalence, mortality, and burden of disease and other adverse health conditions that exist among specific population groups."

Access

We know healthcare access and socioeconomic status make a huge difference in both urban and rural communities. Inadequate access and lower socioeconomic status can cause people to suffer greatly and needlessly. The rates for the five leading causes of death in the U.S. (excluding COVID-19)—heart disease, cancer, unintentional injury (including vehicle accidents and opioid overdoses), chronic lower respiratory disease, and stroke—are higher in poor communities, both rural and urban, as access to adequate, quality healthcare services is limited or nonexistent. And COVID-19 has taken a particularly large toll in these geographic areas. Even with the promise of telehealth to help close the gap, lacking broadband service and the technology to participate means that many people in urban and rural areas still suffer from the "digital divide"—defined as "the gap between people who have access to affordable, reliable internet service (and the skills and gadgets necessary to take advantage of that access) and those who lack it."[1] Digital literacy also continues to be a challenge for those who are poor, older, less educated, and less tech savvy.

Nutrition

The U.S. Department of Agriculture reported 23.5 million people in the U.S. live in "food deserts," where they don't have access to healthy foods like fresh fruits and vegetables; those foods that are available are often highly processed and high in sugar and fats.[2]

"Food swamps"— areas where an abundance of fast food, junk-food outlets, convenience stores, and liquor stores outnumber healthy food options—are also a problem.

And certain segments of the food industry contribute to the poor health and premature deaths of communities without healthy options. Pricing strategies that often make high-fat, high-sugar, highly processed, and nutrient-deficient foods much cheaper than healthy ones, and the bombardment of advertisements, have contributed to an obesity rate of 49.9 percent in the Black adult population and 45.1 percent in Hispanic/Latino adults, compared to an overall obesity rate of 41.9 percent in adults in the U.S.[3] If you live in a poor neighborhood in a major city, a combination of food deserts and food swamps means a greater risk of poor nutrition and a higher rate of obesity as well as the potential health implications, such as conditions like diabetes, heart disease, and cancer.[4]

Housing and Redlining

Beginning in the 1930s, after the Great Depression, redlining emerged as a systemic, discriminatory practice of isolating or steering primarily Black people—who were deemed risky because of their race—to buying or renting housing in certain neighborhoods or buildings. By literally drawing red lines on maps of certain neighborhoods, government-sponsored programs designed a system of segregation by creating predominantly Black neighborhoods. Residents were forced into situations of poor housing with lower real estate values, negatively impacting their ability to create generational wealth. These neighborhoods had insufficient resources to support a healthy lifestyle (food deserts and food swamps), contaminated water, lead paint, electrical line leaks, and climate injustice (e.g., areas with heavy pollution). The result? Health disparities with increased rates of conditions like asthma, cancer, obesity, and lead-related developmental delays that persist today.

While the Fair Housing Act of 1968 was enacted to end this discriminatory practice, its impact has fallen short of solving problems that were baked into the system. These communities have an ongoing legacy of increased risk of premature death, chronic illness, and emotional and mental health conditions, presenting challenges to the health, well-being, and longevity of much of the Black population (and many other people of color).

Financial redlining, the illegal practice of denying a mortgage or imposing a higher interest rate on a loan based on where one lives rather than on the ability to pay, further contributed to these conditions. While this practice of denying financial services to redlined communities was made illegal in 1977, the practice continues to have a negative impact on socioeconomic status and the ability to create generational wealth, which in turn contributes to the health disparities that exist now and for future generations.

Inequities in the Healthcare System

The history of medicine in the U.S. has often been marked by the devastating impacts of systemic racism, sexism, and homophobia. Because of the legacy of such travesties as the U.S. Public Health Service (USPHS) Syphilis Study at Tuskegee, many do not trust the healthcare system. The study, which was conducted from 1932 to 1972, was intended to observe the natural progression of untreated syphilis and involved six hundred African American men as study subjects.[5] There was no informed consent, and antibiotic treatment was not offered, even after it was widely available. (Untreated syphilis can lead to damage to the brain, eyes, heart, nerves, bones, joints, and liver and can result in such complications as paralysis, dementia, and blindness.)

Unfortunately, health disparities continue to be alive and well. COVID-19 has made it clear to many just how severe the repercussions of health inequities can be. Communities of color have been more likely to become infected, to require hospitalization and intubation, and to die.[6] They are also less likely to have access to high-quality healthcare facilities and to receive treatment that can be lifesaving.

The pandemic has brought into stark relief centuries of social, environmental, economic, and political factors that erode the health and shorten the lives of people of color, putting them at higher risk of the chronic conditions that leave immune systems vulnerable to the coronavirus. Many of those same factors fuel the mistrust and fear that leave too many unprotected.

Many people don't have a physician they see regularly, due in part to significant provider shortages, particularly in communities of color, rural areas, and low-income neighborhoods. If they do have a doctor, visits can be too costly even if the patient is insured, particularly if coverage is a high deductible health plan. There are language barriers for those who don't speak English fluently and a fear of deportation among undocumented immigrants. And many providers may not have the necessary expertise to address the unique needs of certain populations, like the LGBTQIA+ community.

Compared to other high-income countries whose life expectancies continued to rise, the overall life expectancy in the U.S. dropped from 78.8 years in 2019 to 76.6 in 2021.[7] And life expectancy in Black and Hispanic communities remains lower than in the white community.

Race/ethnicity

African American women experience a maternal mortality rate that is three to four times greater than their white counterparts, even when educational level and socioeconomic status are equivalent. There is also a disproportionately high mortality rate for Black babies in the

U.S., with 10.8 deaths per thousand live births, compared to a rate of 4.6 for white babies.[8] However, an interesting statistic gleaned from 1.8 million birth records in a Florida hospital between 1992 and 2015 revealed that when Black

HEALTH DISPARITIES[9]

- The low-income, rural Appalachian region has fewer mental health providers and fewer specialty physicians than the rest of the nation—35 percent and 28 percent fewer, respectively—according to the Appalachian Regional Commission (ARC).

- Mental health disparities exist between the sexes; 24.5 percent of women have been diagnosed with a mental illness versus 16.3 percent of men, according to the National Institute of Mental Health (NIMH).

- African Americans suffer the highest mortality rate for all cancers combined, compared with any other racial/ethnic group. African American women have a maternal mortality rate three to four times higher than white women, even when incomes and educational levels are equivalent.

- Approximately 25 percent of Hispanics have high blood pressure. Hispanic women are 40 percent more likely to have cervical cancer and 20 percent more likely to die from cervical cancer than non-Hispanic white women. Puerto Ricans, in particular, "have the highest rate of asthma prevalence compared to any other racial or ethnic group in the U.S.," according to a report from the Asthma and Allergy Foundation of America.[10]

babies were delivered by Black doctors, their mortality rate was cut in half.[11] The research showed no difference in infant mortality with white doctors and white births. Medical literature has indicated that patients with a preference

- Native Americans and Alaska Natives have a higher prevalence of and greater risk factors for mental health and suicide, unintentional injuries, obesity, sudden infant death syndrome (SIDS), diabetes, and liver disease compared to the white population.

- Asian Americans are 40 percent more likely to be diagnosed with diabetes than non-Hispanic white Americans. They are also 80 percent more likely to be diagnosed with end-stage renal disease. Asian Americans are twice as likely to develop chronic hepatitis B than non-Hispanic whites and are eight times more likely to die from hepatitis B than non-Hispanic whites.

- Native Hawaiians and Pacific Islanders have higher rates of smoking, alcohol consumption, and obesity in comparison to other populations, and the incidence rate of tuberculosis is higher than in any other population in the U.S.

- Lesbian and bisexual women have higher rates of breast cancer.[12]

for healthcare providers of the same race/ethnicity, often have better health outcomes and lower associated healthcare costs.[13] Their patient experiences were also more highly rated.[14] (Similar findings have also been observed relative to sex, gender identity, and language.)

According to the U.S. Health and Human Services Office of Minority Health,[15] Native Americans and Alaska Natives frequently contend with issues that impact the ability to access quality medical care and to maximize the pursuit of a healthy lifestyle. These issues include cultural barriers, geographic isolation, inadequate sewage disposal, and low income. Among this population can be found a high prevalence of risk factors for mental health conditions including suicide, unintentional injuries, obesity, substance use, sudden infant death syndrome (SIDS), teenage pregnancy, diabetes, liver disease, and hepatitis.

Among Native Hawaiians and Pacific Islanders, according to the Office of Minority Health, there are higher rates of smoking, alcohol consumption, and obesity. These groups also have less access to cancer prevention and treatment programs. Hepatitis B, HIV/AIDS (human immunodeficiency virus/acquired immunodeficiency syndrome), and tuberculosis are also more prevalent.

Sex/gender/gender identity

Gender bias also exists in the U.S. healthcare system. For example, heart disease is the leading killer of American women, and women die from heart disease at higher rates than men in this country. However, a study in the *Journal of the American Heart Association* found when women receive the same therapies as men, their survival rates are the same.

Often women's complaints are dismissed, or they are told "it's all in your head." A recent study from the University of Miami[16] found that when male and female patients expressed the same amount of pain, female patients were perceived as more likely to benefit from psychotherapy, while medication was more often prescribed for men.

Bias also exists toward the LBGTQIA+ community, and finding adequate access and support can be a challenge. They are often faced with healthcare practitioners who are not as knowledgeable or lack the expertise to address their healthcare needs, which may be unique, such as gender-affirming surgery. Additionally, cultural stigma and discrimination can result in higher rates of mental health disorders, particularly suicide in transgender youth.

Note: We use the acronym LGBTQIA+ to represent the community of individuals who do not identify as cisgender and heterosexual. However, we understand that language continues to evolve to respect and honor everyone as well as to promote and support inclusivity at all times.

Medical Gaslighting

At many points in her life, Carol was subjected to medical gaslighting, with negative and avoidable impacts on her health and well-being, both physical and emotional.

Medical gaslighting is a term appearing more frequently in the press and medical literature. It describes a situation in which a patient's symptoms and concerns are dismissed or trivialized by a healthcare provider, are attributed to stress or hormones, or are viewed as "all in one's head." As a result, the patient may experience a delay—sometimes life threatening—in diagnosis. Patients may doubt themselves, may feel shame or low self-esteem, and may become frustrated by a dismissive healthcare system and the cost of trying to find answers and appropriate treatment.

Medical gaslighting can also occur as a misinterpretation or misdiagnosis of symptoms based on clinical research findings that use a narrowly focused group of patients, typically white men of a certain age. One example is the difference between the symptoms reported by women versus men when they are having a heart attack. Although chest pain is the most common symptom overall, regardless of sex, women may experience different symptoms—including dizziness, nausea and vomiting, heartburn, or unusual and unexplained fatigue—as opposed to the jaw pain, "elephant on the chest," and shortness of breath with which people are more familiar. Consequently, a woman may show up in the ER experiencing a heart attack and be discharged with a GI (gastrointestinal) diagnosis.

Medical gaslighting is reported to be more common in women, communities of color, patients who are obese, those with mental health conditions or disability, those with autoimmune conditions like chronic fatigue syndrome, and the LGBTQIA+ community.

The result? Health disparities persist and these individuals become disillusioned and mistrustful of the healthcare system. Medical gaslighting can create undue stress, anxiety, and depression, and even death in the case of a missed diagnosis, delayed diagnosis, or misdiagnosis. It may also result in an unnecessarily greater cost of care, which impacts out-of-pocket expenses for the patient.

Menopause is a clinical scenario in which medical gaslighting—dismissing or trivializing a woman's symptoms or concerns—may commonly occur. Contributory factors may include gender bias, insufficient medical training and expertise, and a lack of scientific and clinical research.

One of the recurring themes of this book has been the importance of knowing your body and paying attention to changes in your physical and mental health, self-advocacy, asking questions, and standing your ground. Medical gaslighting is yet another reason to take charge of your health and well-being.

The outcomes of your interactions in the healthcare system often depend on your degree of assertiveness, health literacy, and persistence in seeking care from healthcare professionals who are culturally sensitive and display humility, as well as in finding facilities in which staff is trained to meet the needs of a diverse patient population. It is critical to take the time to educate yourself regarding health disparities that may be applicable to your situation and to set expectations regarding (1) having your health issues taken seriously, (2) the need to be informed fully of available options, (3) being alerted to potential side effects, and (4) being treated in the equitable manner we all deserve.

SO, WHAT CAN YOU DO NOW?

- Health disparities can exist due to a variety of factors including age, sex, disability, geographic locale, gender identity, sexual orientation, race/ethnicity, socioeconomic status, education level, and immigrant status. If you believe that a healthcare provider may be biased, racist, and/or dismissive because of your race, ethnicity, age, sex, gender identity, religion, degree of language proficiency, disability, or socioeconomic status, it may ultimately be in your best interest to choose to see someone else, if switching to another provider is possible.

- Health disparities often reflect systemic issues and can negatively impact the way care is delivered, the treatment options offered or not offered, and whether complaints are taken seriously or even ignored. Do not be silent when it comes to your health. Express yourself in an assertive but nonaggressive manner. For example, you might say, "I am not comfortable with the surgery right now. I'd like to talk about other possible treatment options before moving forward." Remember, you have the right to fully understand any medical procedures, along with their benefits and risks, and to give your consent before proceeding. While you may not have a medical background, you know your body best.

- If you are reluctant to speak up or are afraid of being perceived as a difficult patient, you may want a trusted friend or family member to act as your advocate. Your advocate should be prepared to speak on your behalf, ask questions, take notes, and confer with you about next steps. If language is an issue, ask for an interpreter or bring someone with you who can help you fully understand. If in a hospital, there should be a patient relations or social services representative who can address your concerns.

- Do your research, and remember you are the only one who will ever really know how your body feels and what's truly on your mind. Trust your gut. If a clinical interaction does not feel right, a recommendation sounds like it doesn't make sense, or the treatment is not a good fit for your situation, you may well be right. Healthcare professionals are not perfect and all knowing, and you will need to partner with them to successfully manage your individual needs.

- If you believe the quality of care is not what it should be and is due to stereotyping, bias, racism, or sexism, you may want to put your concerns in writing to the provider or business entity. In a hospital, you can bring the matter to the attention of the hospital's administration through a letter or a formal grievance process. And looping in a patient advocate may also be helpful. Remember, you have the right to be treated with respect and dignity and in an equitable manner at all times.

- Seek a second opinion. For conditions like cancer, getting recommendations from another medical professional can be helpful. Identifying medical professionals who speak your preferred language or are familiar with the health beliefs of certain cultures and religions may be key to a better experience and to your overall health and well-being.

- Look for medical professionals with the requisite expertise in culturally sensitive care and a perspective that is inclusive. For some patients, receiving care from a healthcare practitioner of the same race/ethnicity/sex may lead to better outcomes and result in care that is more sensitive to your needs. The following organizations may be helpful in your search:
  - The National Medical Association (NMA)—A professional association of Black/African American physicians focused on parity and justice in medicine and the elimination of disparities in health.

- The Association of American Indian Physicians (AAIP)—A professional physician association focused on American Indian and Alaska Native communities and students.
- The National Council of Asian Pacific Islander Physicians (NCAPIP)—A professional organization of Asian American, Native Hawaiian, and Pacific Islander physicians focused on the advancement of the health and well-being of their patients and communities.
- The National Hispanic Medical Association (NHMA)— A professional organization of Hispanic physicians focused on eliminating health disparities and improving the health of Hispanics.
- GLMA--A professional organization of health professionals focused on ensuring the equality in healthcare for LGBTQIA+ individuals and healthcare professionals.
- Health in Her Hue—A new company that provides a digital platform connecting Black women and women of color to culturally competent healthcare providers, health content, and an online community.
- OutCare Health—A ". . . comprehensive resource for LGBTQ+ healthcare, including provider and healthcare resource directories, mentorship, medical education reform, and cultural competency training. The OutList is an online, nationwide directory of healthcare providers who identify as culturally competent in the care of the LGBTQ+ community."[17]

CHAPTER 11

Paying for Healthcare

No parent should ever have to decide if they can afford to save their child's life. It just shouldn't happen. Not here.

JIMMY KIMMEL

JOE'S STORY

Joe, age fifty-five, had been the director of learning and development for a company in Maryland for nineteen years. In March 2020, he was furloughed, along with many other company employees, as a result of the COVID-19 pandemic. His wife, fifty-three, a contractor for a travel agency specializing in cruise vacations, lost her job as well.

Joe applied for unemployment and received his benefits, plus a $600 per week government supplement until July 31st. As a contractor rather than an employee, his wife was originally ineligible for all unemployment benefits. In mid-May 2020, she was eventually accepted into the Pandemic

Unemployment Assistance (PUA) program, receiving the minimum allowable unemployment benefits.

Through his employer, Joe had family medical coverage—including dental and vision—for his wife and two daughters, ages twenty-two and twenty-four, who had planned to stay on their father's insurance until age twenty-six. Their older daughter, an education specialist for the local school system, was not eligible for benefits from her employer. Their younger daughter, working from home as a marketing manager, had a company-sponsored health insurance program available to her. However, because this program was costly for a young adult just starting out in her career, she originally opted to stay on her family's insurance plan.

Although the furlough took place in March 2020, Joe's company's health insurance was extended until the first week of June. With the continued downturn of business due to the pandemic, Joe's benefits were finally suspended. With help from his company, Joe was offered COBRA (Consolidated Omnibus Budget Reconciliation Act) health insurance for eighteen months, but now that he was unemployed, the cost of COBRA family coverage was just too steep.

Joe then investigated Maryland's Health Exchange website, established by the Affordable Care Act (ACA) in 2010. Determining which plan was affordable was a difficult task because of their 2019 income tax bracket. Although advertised as "affordable," Joe's family did not qualify for any level of insurance he could afford. With no regular income, even the lowest-cost, high-deductible plans ($870 per month, with a $7,900 deductible) were too expensive given the family's financial resources.

A health insurance broker and a financial planner were enlisted to help Joe find cost-effective health insurance for his now very financially strained family. The health insurance broker confirmed what he already knew—to pay for the lowest coverage available, he would be forced to withdraw funds from his 401(k) plan, which was earmarked for retirement.

Throughout the year, Joe's family continued to work daily to find solutions to their financial crisis due to the pandemic.

Joe's elder daughter discovered if she were to complete her 2019 taxes as an individual rather than as a dependent of her parents, she might qualify for a low-cost Medicaid program. She amended her taxes to reflect this change and applied for Medicaid. Fortunately, she was accepted.

Joe's younger daughter applied and received company-sponsored insurance four years earlier than planned. These insurance premiums created an additional financial burden, as she had to use money earmarked for her college loan repayment.

Joe and his family withdrew funds from his 401(k) plan to pay for healthcare and other basic living expenses. Both Joe and his wife continued to seek employment and to take extra precautions to maintain their health.

At the beginning of 2021, Joe and his wife applied for and received health insurance coverage at a cost of $95.30 per month. However, after they filed their 2020 taxes in April, the cost was reduced to $6.94 per month due to their lack of income in 2020. Joe realized that affordable coverage is possible, but, if you lose employer-sponsored coverage at the beginning of the year, you may have to wait almost an entire year to qualify for more affordable coverage. It is sad that many people without affordable coverage are forced to choose food and rent over medical care.

LESSONS LEARNED

- When he lost his employer-sponsored healthcare coverage, Joe realized how difficult it can be to find affordable insurance. To reduce the stress and anxiety of figuring out how to pay for healthcare expenses due to an unforeseen medical condition or accident, Joe had to learn, as quickly as possible, what options were available.

- Joe's resourcefulness led him to learn more about the plans offered as a result of the Affordable Care Act (ACA) and through Medicaid, in addition to seeking the services of a health insurance broker and financial planner.

WHAT YOU NEED TO KNOW

Joe's story is unfortunately all too common. Millions of people in the U.S. face this healthcare affordability issue, which has been further exacerbated by the COVID-19 pandemic. According to the Office of Health Policy, 29.2 million people in the country lacked healthcare coverage in 2021, down from 31.1 million.[1] A 2021 Federal Reserve report indicated 11 percent of Americans would not be able to pay an unexpected $400 expense, and 8 percent would need to borrow from a friend or family member or sell something to cover the cost.[2]

A 2022 survey conducted by the Kaiser Family Foundation[3] found that 100 million Americans (41 percent of adults) are living with healthcare debt. The report also indicated approximately one in seven people with debt had been denied access to care due to unpaid bills, and approximately 66 percent delayed care because of the cost. Medical expenses are number one on the list of contributing factors leading to bankruptcies by individuals each year.[4]

While the Affordable Care Act (ACA) of 2010 provided healthcare options to people who were not eligible through Medicaid, Medicare, or an employer, the cost of healthcare insurance has continued to remain out of reach for many Americans. And the residents of states in the U.S. that refused to expand Medicaid have been hit even harder. Unfortunately, many of those states already had high rates of poverty and low-income households.

> **TOP FIVE HEALTHCARE ISSUES MOST IMPORTANT TO CONSUMERS***
>
> 1 Having affordable insurance options
> 2 Out-of-pocket healthcare costs
> 3 Cost of health insurance premiums
> 4 Cost of prescription drugs
> 5 Cost of hospital care
>
> *Consumer Perspectives on Patient Experience in the U.S. The Beryl Institute Ipsos PX Pulse Survey. December 2021.

Healthcare spending in the United States ranks the highest of any developed country in the world. (See the sidebar on the next page for a comparison with other countries.) In 2020, national spending on healthcare goods and services was $4.01 trillion, or 18 percent of GDP (gross domestic product). On average, the U.S. spends twice as much on healthcare per person compared to other developed countries.[5]

The High Cost of Healthcare

Why are healthcare costs so high in the U.S.? The costs are mostly driven by higher payments to hospitals and physicians, higher costs of prescription drugs, and administrative costs. The aging population, along with high rates of obesity and chronic disease, also contribute. Many developed countries have a government-sponsored healthcare system for their citizens, similar to Medicare, that negotiates prices and manages payments. If healthcare was covered as a right, not based on employment status or the personal ability to pay, there would be a greater likelihood that people would be able to seek medical attention earlier, stay healthier, and avoid more expensive hospitalizations, thereby reducing the cost of care.

While we spend more money on healthcare in the U.S., our health outcomes and quality of care are worse compared to many other developed countries. Life expectancy in the U.S. ranks twenty-eighth out of the thirty-six OECD (Organization for Economic Co-operation and Development) countries. In fact, U.S. life expectancy decreased from 78.8 years in 2019 to 76.1 in 2021.[7] Infant mortality is thirty-third out of the

COUNTRIES SPENDING THE MOST ON HEALTHCARE ($ PER CAPITA)[6]

- United States ($10,948)
- Switzerland ($7,138)
- Norway ($6,748)
- Germany ($6,731)
- Netherlands ($6,299)
- Austria ($5,899)
- Denmark ($5,849)
- Sweden ($5,754)
- Ireland ($5,604)
- France ($5,564)

thirty-six OECD nations, and the U.S. is the only industrialized nation in the world where maternal mortality is rising.[8] The chronic diseases among U.S. adults—heart disease, diabetes, hypertension, and depression—rank the highest, with an obesity rate two times higher than the OECD average.[9]

Additionally, medical debt is a top reason for personal bankruptcy in the U.S., and it also has risen during the pandemic. According to a Kaiser Family Foundation analysis,[10] it is more common among those aged thirty-five to sixty-four, who are more likely to be in debt than other age groups. Those with Medicare coverage were the least likely. Medical debt was more common in women than men, and those with income under $50,000 were four times more likely to have medical debt than those with an income over $75,000. 16 percent of Black adults had medical debt, compared to 9 percent in white and Hispanic populations.

When you go into medical debt and cannot keep up with payments, you will likely deal with a collection agency and have your credit rating negatively impacted. Your poor credit rating can result in higher rates of interest on other loans, like the purchase of a car or getting a mortgage, or not being eligible for a loan at all. In the past, even if you paid off your medical debt, it might remain on your credit report and lower your credit score. Beginning July 2022, three national credit reporting agencies—Transunion, Experian, and Equifax—changed their policies regarding unpaid medical debt.[11] Medical debt will not appear on credit reports until it is twelve months old (up from six months) or if it is less than $500.

How much does your healthcare cost?

Unlike many other purchases, most people do not know the charges for medical care before being treated. When medical procedures are elective, we may be more apt to shop around. More often, we are in distress, perhaps experiencing pain, and just want to feel better no matter what it takes. Rarely do we ask in advance how much a procedure or surgery is going to cost, and we are reluctant to even raise the concern. Those most likely to inquire are those without coverage and often in the greatest need of care. When they find out, and the choice is between medical care or feeding the family and paying the rent, medical care is the most likely choice to be deferred. In many cases, the healthcare practitioner providing your care may not even know the cost and will refer you to the billing department. Often, we are surprised when we get the final bill. If a hospital bill is itemized, we see the shocking charges for each pill, IV fluids, dressings, etc.

Prices can vary widely from one hospital, healthcare facility, lab, and practitioner to another, even in the same geographical area. Most people, however, go to the nearest medical office/facility or see the provider recommended by others, without knowing what the charges will be. In addition, some actions may not be medically necessary, and you may want to question whether the procedure is needed.

A new Hospital Price Transparency ruling was officially enacted in January 2021, with a plan for phased implementation through 2024. This federal rule requires hospitals to make public, through a machine-readable digital file, its standard charges for all items and services, to help prevent surprises after a hospital procedure and reduce the financial risk for both the hospital and the patient. This includes any negotiated rates with health plans and any discounted rates for cash. The ruling also requires hospitals to post online the costs of three hundred "shoppable" procedures, along with an explanation of each, to create more pricing competition among hospitals, as patients may want to shop for the best price for a medical procedure.

However, the Departments of Labor (DOL), Health and Human Services (HHS), and the Treasury collectively announced they would defer enforcement. The departments also explained they would delay indefinitely the requirement to publish negotiated rates for prescription drugs. The bottom line? At the time of publication of this book, many hospitals have not complied with the legislation. Full hospital cost transparency will clearly take longer than initially planned, and consumers will need to make requests for the information they need and advocate hard to obtain it.

Employer-Sponsored Health Insurance

More than 50 percent of the U.S. population purchases health insurance through their place of employment. Thus, losing one's job can become a disastrous situation for individuals and families.

An employer typically buys a group plan with an insurance company at a negotiated rate for its employees. By purchasing a fully insured group plan, the company pays a flat rate to the health insurance company to process the claims and handle all the administrative duties and expenses. The company's employees must adhere to the insurer's coverage policies, network of providers, and preset case management services. That group rate can vary widely across the country, but generally, the larger—and younger and healthier—the size of the group, the greater the discount that can be negotiated.

However, many large companies are *self-insured*, which means the company is assuming the financial risk of paying for the health claims themselves, while a third-party administrator may be hired to process the claims according to the company's benefit plan. Self-insured plans give the company the opportunity to customize their plan to meet employee needs and likely save the company money on premium costs. With a self-insured plan, the company's benefits staff and/or executive may act as the final arbiter in any claim disputes or appeals.

Whether your employer's health benefit coverage is fully insured or self-insured, companies and health insurers continue to seek ways to contain the growing increase in U.S. healthcare costs. Depending on the number of claims and the cost of care delivered to employees and their dependents, many of these rising costs may be passed onto the employee population as part of their healthcare premium increases each year, along with any changes to the plan's coverage levels.

At the end of each plan year, your employer and the insurance company will review the cost of healthcare claims paid that year to determine how much to charge employees to cover the projected claims for the coming year. An employer will typically charge its employees a subsidized rate for the cost of "employee-only" coverage and will charge more for "employee +1" and "family" coverage. The average annual premium for a family of four was $22,221 in 2021, but employers picked up 73 percent of the cost. The average annual premium for a single employee in 2021 was $7,739.11.[12]

Know How Your Insurance Plan Works

In Chapter 2, we discussed the importance of knowing before you get sick what your health insurance plan covers, to help avoid surprises. You also need to know how much you will have to pay out-of-pocket before the insurance kicks in. This amount can vary greatly, so it's important to know how your plan works and to select the option that will work best for you each year. Remember, just because your healthcare practitioner orders a test, medication, or procedure, it does not necessarily mean your health plan will cover it. If there is any question, your practitioner or you should contact the insurance company to find out if there are any steps that must be taken for review and approval of requested services before they are rendered (called 'prior authorization').

HMO (health maintenance organization) vs. PPO (preferred provider organization)

Your employer may offer different types of health insurance plans. If cost is most important to you, you may want to consider choosing an HMO (health maintenance organization). HMO plans typically have lower monthly premiums and out-of-pocket costs. However, HMOs only provide care within a designated network of providers. If you don't select a healthcare provider within the network and go out-of-network, the service is not covered (unless in cases of an emergency where access to the network is not available). Also, HMOs typically require a referral from a PCP (primary care practitioner) before scheduling with a specialist in the network. Typically, you don't need to file a claim, as the HMOs pay the network providers directly.

PPO (preferred provider organization) plans generally have higher monthly premiums but allow you the flexibility to seek medical care both in and out-of-network. If it is important to you to have the option of seeing any healthcare provider you want, without a referral, then a PPO might work best. However, if you do go out-of-network, you will pay more and may have a separate deductible or co-pay. In some cases, you may have to pay the out-of-network doctor and file a claim with the insurance company to get reimbursed, because healthcare practitioners who are not contracted with your health insurance company have no obligation to submit claims on your behalf.

High deductible health plan (HDHP)

In 2020, 52.9 percent of employees in the U.S. with insurance through their employer had coverage through a high deductible health plan.[13] An HDHP is defined by the IRS for 2022 as any medical plan with a deductible of at least $1,400 for an individual ($2,800 for a family) and a total yearly out-of-pocket expense (including deductibles, co-payments, and coinsurance) that is no more than $7,050 for an individual (or $14,100 for a family). The limit does not apply to out-of-network services.

An HDHP can be paired with a health savings account (HSA), which allows certain medical expenses to be paid from what you contribute to the account, and the money in the account is not subject to federal taxes.

Health Insurance Plan Terminology

Here are some common terms associated with health insurance plans. While it can seem like a foreign language, it's important to learn what they mean and to understand how your plan works:

Open Enrollment—the time each year during which you can select the type of plan that will best suit your needs in the upcoming year. It is also a chance to add or delete coverage to a plan that is being renewed. Once open enrollment ends, it is typically not possible to make any changes until the next year, except in the case of certain qualifying events, like divorce or marriage, birth, or adoption of a child.

Deductible—a specified amount of money you must pay out-of-pocket before insurance coverage will kick in. Some plans have separate deductibles for certain services like prescription drugs.

One way to contain costs is to choose a high-deductible plan. These plans have lower monthly premiums but do not pay for covered medical expenses until a certain dollar amount of healthcare costs is incurred and paid by you. In 2022, these deductibles typically ranged from $1,400 to $6,900 for an individual, and from $2,800 to $13,800 for family coverage.[14] So, while these high-deductible insurance plans keep the monthly payments for coverage itself low, people may be hit with a huge upfront medical expense in the event of an accident or emergency, as well as with expensive medications.

Many high deductible plans cover certain preventive care services like mammograms and annual checkups at 100 percent, so there would be no out-of-pocket costs for them. It is important to find out if your plan offers such coverage. Finances can often cause people to skip or put off annual checkups, routine cancer screenings, immunizations, prescribed medications, and other preventive services. These actions are the very things, along with a healthy lifestyle (a nutritious diet, regular physical activity, ample sleep, stress and weight management, etc.) and the management of chronic conditions, that help optimize your health and well-being. In turn, a healthier population means lower costs for all, as well the additional cost savings for you as an individual that may be achieved by early detection of health problems, reduction of the impact of chronic conditions, and seeking care in the most appropriate setting.

Co-pay—A co-pay is the predetermined amount you pay each time for a healthcare service. For example, you may pay a $25 co-pay every time you visit your physician, or a $250 co-pay each time you go to the emergency room. Co-pays typically do not count toward your deductible, so even if you've reached the deductible amount, you will still have the co-pays.

Coinsurance—Coinsurance is the percentage of costs you pay versus your health plan for covered services after you've met your benefit period deductible. For example, suppose your health insurance plan's allowed amount for an office visit is $100, and your coinsurance is 20 percent. If you've paid your deductible, you pay $20, and the insurance plan covers the rest. However, if you haven't met your deductible, you must pay the full $100.

Out-of-pocket maximum—In your health insurance plan, you will want to find out the specific out-of-pocket maximum, as this is the most you will spend out-of-pocket in the benefit plan year, not including your monthly premiums. Most plans run from January through December each year. But some use a different twelve-month time period.

After the out-of-pocket maximum is reached, the insurance will pay 100 percent of the covered medical expenses. Remember, you still must pay your monthly premiums. These amounts can vary from one plan to another and may be adjusted from one year to the next.

Usual and customary (U&C) charges (sometimes referred to as reasonable and customary [R&C], or usual and prevailing [U&P] charges)—Most insurance companies will have determined a reasonable charge they will pay for each service based on the prevailing costs of that service within a specified geographical area. So, for example, a knee replacement procedure will likely cost more in New York City than in Topeka, Kansas. However, a physician may charge more than the usual and prevailing rate and may charge you for any amount that your insurance does not cover (if the provider is out-of-network). So, ask how much the procedure is going to cost and how much your insurance will cover, to avoid any surprises.

Explanation of benefits (EOB)—An EOB (explanation of benefits) is a statement from your health insurance plan that outlines the charges for your care after a claim has been submitted by your provider. It identifies the service(s) covered by your health insurance plan, how much your health plan will pay, and how much you are responsible for paying. The coverage amounts depend on your type of plan; your co-pay or coinsurance levels; the amount of discount, if any, the health plan has been able to negotiate with the provider; and if you have reached your deductible or out-of-pocket maximum for the plan year. When you receive a bill from your provider, be sure to compare it to the EOB to ensure you pay the correct amount, if any, that is your responsibility under your benefit plan.

Coordination of benefits (COB)—Coordination of benefits is the process used when a patient has insurance coverage involving more than one entity. Typically, there are rules that determine which entity pays first (primary coverage) and entities that have an obligation to pay some or all of the remaining costs (secondary and Medigap coverage). The rules may differ for those with commercial health plan coverage as the main insurance compared to Medicare and/or Medicaid. Coordination of benefits may also involve other types of insurance than medical insurance. One example would be auto insurance in the case of injuries due to a car accident. In such a scenario, your car insurance may pay first and then go to your medical insurance carrier to be reimbursed for any costs the auto carrier considers to be outside the scope of the policy and to be the responsibility of the medical carrier. An auto insurer may also go to the insurer of the other party involved in the accident.

Tax-Saving Plan Features

Some employer plans include features that provide tax savings for you. Generally, you can opt into these features based on your personal or family situation.

Flexible spending account (FSA)—If you have health insurance coverage through your employer, you may be offered a flexible spending account (FSA) to hold funds for paying co-payments, deductibles, and eligible drug and healthcare costs. Setting aside a certain amount of FSA money on a pretax basis can help reduce your taxable income.

There is an annual contribution limit established by the IRS as well as a list of potentially eligible medical and drug expenses. However, your employer may limit the types of expenses for which your FSA can be used. Eligible expenses may vary, so it is important to check first before assuming you will be able to use FSA funds.

It is important to estimate your out-of-pocket eligible expenses for the coming year and not put in more money than you think you'll need. Generally, you cannot "roll over" funds from one year to the next. If you do not spend all the money you contributed within the plan year, it will not be available to you in the next year. However, in special circumstances, your employer may decide to make an exception and extend the time frame or carry over a predetermined maximum amount to the coming year. Some employers did so for the 2020 plan year because of the COVID-19 pandemic.

Health savings account (HSA)—Some employers may offer a benefit called a health savings account (HSA) to help pay for out-of-pocket eligible medical expenses on a pretax basis. An HSA cannot exist as a stand-alone account. It must be paired with a high deductible health plan.

You determine how much money to put into the account each year during annual enrollment, up to a limit established by the IRS. HSA funds do not have a "use-it-or-lose-it" provision. Therefore, any money contributed but not spent generally can roll over from year to year. These dollars typically cannot be used to pay health insurance premiums but can be used to cover expenses (on a list defined each year by the IRS) that may not be covered by your insurance plan. The before-tax feature is a good benefit because it lowers your taxable income in each year that you make a contribution.

If you are insured through your workplace, your employer can also contribute (up to an annual limit determined by the IRS) but is not obligated to do so. There is an IRS-defined annual limit for the combination of contributions made by the employee and the employer. You will want to find out how to take advantage of this benefit if you have sufficient discretionary dollars available.

Health reimbursement account (HRA)—A health reimbursement account is a way for employers to reimburse employees on a pretax basis for qualified medical expenses incurred by the employee or their dependents.

As with HSAs and FSAs, the list of items eligible for coverage may vary from year to year. And the size of the account may also vary each year based on employer and/or governmental regulations.

There are several rules that currently apply to HRAs:

- HRAs must be funded entirely by the employer, so nothing is deducted from the employee's paycheck, and the contribution made by the employer is not counted in the employee's income.

- Unlike FSAs and HSAs, there's no upper limit on how much employers can contribute to *individual* HRAs and no minimum contribution requirements. However, there are certain rules which the employer must follow.

- If traditional group health insurance is offered, employers can offer a second type of HRA called an *excepted benefit* HRA.[15] Employees can enroll in an excepted benefit HRA even if they are not on their employer's health plan. They can use the money in the HRA to pay for short-term health insurance, qualified medical expenses, and vision and dental premiums, but not purchase comprehensive health insurance. (In 2023, these plans reimburse employees for up to $1,950 for qualified medical expenses.)

- Although the IRS defines what constitutes a qualified medical expense, employers can further limit the expenses eligible for reimbursement.

- To be reimbursed, you must provide documentation of the expense and that it meets eligibility criteria.

- In most cases, you cannot have both an HRA and an HSA.

The rules governing FSA, HSA, and HRA accounts can be complicated and can change over time. It is important you stay up to date and take the time to understand them, each health plan year. If you have questions, don't hesitate to ask your manager or human resources/benefits representative.

Dental Insurance

Some dental work—such as crowns, root canals, and implants—can be very expensive, and you may be interested in purchasing dental insurance. However, before enrolling in your employer-sponsored dental insurance plan or obtaining dental insurance on your own, you'll want to investigate what the plan covers and how it works, to determine whether it is cost-effective for you.

There are several considerations:

- First, if the dental insurance involves a preferred provider organization (PPO) or dental health maintenance organization (DHMO), you will want to check to see if your dentist is in the network. Depending on the plan, you may pay more for your dental care out-of-pocket if your dentist is not in the network or if you are not willing to switch to an in-network dentist.

- What is the annual maximum the dental plan will pay? Some dental insurance plans have an annual limit of $1,000 or $1,500, which may not cover more expensive treatment.

- If you typically get one or two exams and cleanings each year, will the monthly premiums, deductible, and coinsurance or co-pay add up to more than you would pay out-of-pocket?

- Check to see if there is a waiting period if you need more-extensive dental work. Some plans may require a three- or six-month waiting period before covering more expensive procedures.

- Review the specifics of what the plan covers. For example, orthodontics, for children and adults, may be limited or not included at all. Cosmetic dentistry procedures, such as teeth whitening, are generally not covered.

As with any insurance, it's important to understand what you're paying for and to decide what's right for your situation.

Prescription Drugs

The cost of medications continues to increase and can be financially challenging, particularly if you have a chronic condition, are on several different medicines, and/or need specialty pharmacy meds (such as an injection or infusion for conditions like immune disorders, genetic enzyme deficiencies, or certain cancer treatments).

According to the Health Policy Institute (2021), about two-thirds or 66 percent of U.S. adults take prescription drugs.[16]

And, on average, the older you are, the greater the number of medications you likely are taking.

If you have coverage for prescription drugs through an employer plan, the type and degree of coverage will vary by employer and by health plan. For example, some plans provide 100 percent coverage for medications for chronic conditions like hypertension and diabetes. In some instances, your out-of-pocket co-pay/coinsurance contributions may apply to an overall deductible. However, in other cases, there may be a deductible for medical services and a separate deductible for medications.

Those eligible for Medicare have access to Medicare Part D for drug coverage. Patients who are members of a Medicare Advantage Plan (also called Medicare Part C or MA plan) typically have medication coverage included.

Spending time comparison shopping can pay off when it comes to medications. The cost of the exact same medication in the exact same dose may vary from pharmacy to pharmacy in the exact same geographic location. Additionally, sometimes paying out-of-pocket may be cheaper than using insurance coverage, depending on the medication. For example, sometimes the cost of a drug may be lower than your co-pay or coinsurance. If you do not anticipate reaching your annual deductible, this may be the less expensive way to go; however, paying without using your insurance means those amounts will not count toward your deductible.

There are several potential ways to save money on prescription drugs, depending on whether you have insurance coverage, the provisions of the insurance plan, and the type of medications you take. It is important for you to find out the rules for each, depending on your situation. Some options potentially available to lower the cost of drugs include but are not limited to the following:

- Discount cards—Discount percent varies depending on the card and medication
- 90-day supply—Can be helpful when you are on the same medication and dosage on an ongoing basis
- Mail order—Often combined with a 90-day supply
- Generics instead of brand name drugs—Applicable for some medications
- Drug manufacturer discounts and coupons—Varies by manufacturer for certain medications
- Health insurance companies
- State/local programs and community health centers
- New resources like Cost Plus Drug Company—Drugs offered at cost plus 15 percent

COBRA

According to COBRA (Consolidated Omnibus Budget Reconciliation Act), established in 1985, you may be able to elect to continue your employer-sponsored health coverage if you lose coverage due to any of the following:

- You quit your job.
- You were fired, unless it was for "gross misconduct."
- Your hours were reduced.
- You lost coverage because of a death, divorce, or legal separation.

However, COBRA coverage is expensive, as you now have to pay the full amount of the premium—both the employer's portion and yours—plus a 2 percent administrative fee.

COBRA coverage is not automatic; you have sixty days to enroll, and it is retroactive. The coverage can last up to eighteen months for the employee and can be stopped if other insurance is obtained. For a spouse or dependent children, the coverage can last up to thirty-six months.

Be sure to also check out your health insurance plan options under the Affordable Care Act (ACA) in your state.

Medicare and Medicare Advantage

Medicare is our country's health insurance program for people ages sixty-five or older. You're first eligible to sign up for Medicare three months before you turn sixty-five. Certain people who are younger than sixty-five may also qualify if they have certain conditions, such as end-stage renal disease (ESRD) and need dialysis or a kidney transplant, or ALS (amyotrophic lateral sclerosis, also known as Lou Gehrig's disease). To qualify if you are under sixty-five, you need to have received Social Security Disability Insurance (SSDI) checks for at least twenty-four months.

There are specific eligibility requirements and periods when you can enroll in Medicare plans. Go to medicare.gov to see if you meet them and when you should be taking action. If you don't enroll when you're first eligible for Medicare, you could be subject to a late-enrollment penalty.

Medicare plans have several different parts:

- Part A covers inpatient hospital care, skilled nursing facility care, hospice care, nursing home care (inpatient care in a skilled nursing facility that's not custodial or long-term care), and home healthcare.

- Part B covers services deemed to be medically necessary and preventive care services; includes physician services, outpatient care, ambulance services, durable medical equipment, limited outpatient prescription drugs, clinical research (certain qualifying studies), and mental health services.

- Parts A and B are considered to be traditional or Original Medicare, in which doctors and hospitals get paid for services rendered.

- Part C includes Medicare Advantage plans (or MA plans), which are another way to get your Medicare Parts A and B coverage through government-approved private companies that must follow the rules set by Medicare. Some MA plans offer additional benefits such as dental, vision, and hearing aids.

- Part D helps cover the cost of prescription drugs. If you are enrolled in Original Medicare, Part D can be purchased as a stand-alone plan through private companies. Part D benefits may be included in a Medicare Advantage Plan.

According to the Kaiser Family Foundation, roughly 42 percent of Medicare recipients are enrolled in a Medicare Advantage Plan.[17] A Medicare Advantage Plan may be an HMO, PPO, private fee-for-service plan, or a Special Needs Plan (SNP). A Medicare SNP is designed to serve only people diagnosed with a particular chronic condition, such as congestive heart failure. The plan might include access to a specialized network of providers and may feature clinical case management programs designed to serve the special needs of people with this condition.

Private Medicare plans have pre-negotiated rates with healthcare practitioners who are deemed in-network. You will want to ask your healthcare provider if s/he accepts Medicare reimbursement without charging you the balance of their fees.

MEDICARE & END-STAGE RENAL DISEASE (ESRD)

End-stage renal disease (ESRD) is kidney disease severe enough that your kidneys no longer work and you require ongoing dialysis, or you have had a kidney transplant. Medicare provides coverage for the cost of care if you meet eligibility requirements. You should contact Medicare to ensure you qualify.

If you have ESRD, you can select either Original Medicare or a Medicare Advantage Plan (Part C). To get the full benefits available under Medicare to cover certain dialysis and kidney transplant services, you'll need to sign up for both Part A (hospital insurance) and Part B (medical insurance). If you are eligible for coverage of ESRD by Medicare, you will be required to have prescription drug coverage equivalent to Medicare's basic prescription drug plan (Part D).

You will want to choose carefully, depending on your needs and eligibility, budget, and the level of flexibility in choosing the healthcare providers you want. Each year, during the Medicare open enrollment period, you can evaluate the benefits of your current plan and compare it with other options that may be available to you. For more information about Medicare, go to medicare.gov.

Medicaid

Medicaid is a joint federal and state program that can provide health coverage for people with limited income and resources, including *some* families, and children, pregnant women, the elderly, and people with disabilities. Medicaid may also cover eligible skilled nursing services, rehabilitation, and long-term care provided by certified nursing homes. Medicaid is administered at the state level following federal guidelines.

Depending on the state in which you reside, your annual income must be below a specified amount to qualify for Medicaid. Additional factors like household size, disability, and family status may impact eligibility criteria. Eligibility requirements may vary significantly from state to state and may change from year to year. Coverage may also change from year to year. To see if you are eligible, visit your state's Medicaid website, Medicaid.gov, and HHS.gov for more information.

Dual Eligibles—Dually eligible beneficiaries are individuals enrolled in both Medicare and Medicaid who are eligible by virtue of their age or disability and low incomes and meet the requirements for Medicare and Medicaid. They are enrolled in Medicare Part A and/or Part B and in full-benefit Medicaid and/or the Medicare Savings Programs (MSPs), which are administered by each individual state and assist low-income Medicare beneficiaries with some or all Part A and B expenses.

The Affordable Care Act (ACA)

According to the American Medical Association, "The Affordable Care Act (ACA) is a comprehensive reform law, enacted in 2010, that increases health insurance coverage for the uninsured and implements reforms to the health insurance market."[18]

The ACA increased the number of people eligible for healthcare coverage, including dependent children up to age twenty-six, brought greater focus to preventive care, and provided coverage for preexisting conditions that may have been previously denied. It made changes to the reimbursement system for healthcare providers, including hospitals and physicians, with a goal of lowering cost and increasing quality.

ACA plans are available to those meeting the eligibility criteria. As always in healthcare, it is important to understand your options and decide the best path for you.

The Children's Health Insurance Program (CHIP)[19]

The Children's Health Insurance Program (CHIP) "provides low-cost health coverage to children in families that earn too much to qualify for Medicaid. In some states, CHIP also covers pregnant women. Each state offers CHIP coverage and works closely with its state Medicaid program. Like Medicaid, the rules and eligibility requirements can vary from state to state."

TRICARE[20]

TRICARE is "the uniformed services health care program for active-duty service members (ADSMs), active-duty family members (ADFMs), National Guard and Reserve members and their family members, retirees and retiree family members, survivors, and certain former spouses worldwide." Care is available through the Military Health System (MHS), a global, integrated system that includes military hospitals or clinics, a civilian network of providers, or TRICARE-authorized non-network providers.

Disability Insurance

Disability insurance provides a portion of your income (generally up to 60 percent) if you are sick and/or injured and unable to work. Depending on your policy, it may apply if you cannot work at all or if you can no longer perform the duties of your job in your specific area of training or expertise. For example, a surgeon who has developed a severe tremor or severely impaired vision and therefore is no longer able to perform surgery may be eligible.

There are two types of disability coverage—short-term disability (STD) and long-term disability (LTD)—depending on the length of the disability. The eligibility criteria and the duration of the coverage may vary depending on the policy and the company. If you have the option to purchase a group policy from your employer, it is typically less expensive than an individual policy. However, it is important to do your research and determine the best coverage for your situation within the scope of your financial means. Generally, the older you are, the more expensive disability insurance becomes. If you delay too long, you may find you may not meet the eligibility criteria, or a policy may become cost prohibitive.

Additionally, there are two federal programs—Social Security Disability Insurance (SSDI) and Supplemental Security Income (SSI). SSDI may be available in situations of disability after earning enough Social Security work credits within a certain time. Under certain circumstances, SSDI may be available to a spouse or former spouse and children. SSI is not the same as Social Security and is not funded by Social Security. It is intended for older adults (generally sixty-five and older) with a disability, who have limited or no income and resources. There are specific eligibility criteria for each program.

Long-Term Care (LTC) Insurance

According to the U.S. Department of Health and Human Services' Administration for Community Living, 70 percent of those who are sixty-five and older will likely need some long-term care services at some point. Long-term care (LTC) insurance provides coverage for a variety of services that are typically not covered by health insurance. These services may include assistance with activities of daily living such as bathing, dressing, or eating, the help of a health aide or caregiver, or home modifications (e.g., wheelchair ramp). The need for long-term care may be critical in situations like dementia, disability, or a debilitating chronic condition.

Like disability insurance, the amount of coverage, the range of services, and duration of the coverage may vary by policy and by company and is generally cheaper if you are able to purchase it as part of a group plan through an employer. You typically have options regarding waiting periods, levels of service coverage, and applicable care settings (e.g., home vs. nursing home), all of which impact the cost of the premium.

As with disability insurance, the older you are, the more expensive the coverage. Notwithstanding the negative impact of COVID-19, overall longevity has generally increased over time, and more people are using their long-term care coverage and for an extended period of time. Delaying the purchase of long-term care insurance may result in a policy which is cost prohibitive or no longer available.

If You Are Self-Employed

Finding insurance coverage if you are self-employed can be challenging and often makes those interested in having their own business take pause. Here are some possibilities:

- If you are transitioning from an employer that offered health insurance, you may be eligible for COBRA coverage for eighteen months.

- ACA (Affordable Care Act) coverage through the Health Insurance Marketplace is another option.

- If your business has even one employee (other than yourself, a spouse, family member, or owner), you may be able to use the SHOP (Small Business Health Options Program) Marketplace for small businesses to offer coverage to yourself and your employees.

- Depending on your financial circumstances, you may be eligible for Medicaid, the health insurance program intended for those with limited financial means. Medicaid operates as a joint effort between the federal government and the states. As such, the plans can vary widely from state to state.

- Section 1331 of the Affordable Care Act gives states the option of creating a Basic Health Program (BHP), providing coverage for low-income residents whose income fluctuates above and below the Medicaid and CHIP levels. Check to see if your state offers this type of plan.

Filing Claims and Claim Appeals

In most cases, your doctor's office and hospital will submit the insurance claims for you. However, if you're out-of-network and have to pay the bill yourself, you may need to file the claim on your own. Generally, there's a claim form on your insurance company's website, or you may be able to obtain one from your employer. You will need to include all the pertinent information—policy number, name of patient covered under your plan, whether you have other insurance, and if this was due to a work-related incident or car accident. You will want to include all doctor bills listing what treatment was provided and all receipts. Many plans have deadlines for submitting claims (usually sixty or ninety days), so you will want to submit the claim promptly.

Claims can be denied for a variety of reasons, including but not limited to:

- The service is not covered by your plan
- The service is deemed to be not medically necessary or experimental/investigational
- Lack of prior authorization from the insurance company
- Missing or incorrect information
- Coding error by the physician
- Submission is too late

The health plan will offer an appeals process if you believe the claim was valid and unfairly denied. You will want to gather the requisite information to substantiate your appeal, which could include a letter from your physician or perhaps an explanation of why the treatment was needed. Your practitioner can also appeal on your behalf. Depending on the insurance plan, you (or a representative on your behalf) and your practitioner can appeal your case with an appeals committee.

Be persistent. According to a March 2022 Medscape Medical News article, less than 1 percent (0.2 percent, to be exact) of claims denials are appealed by patients, even though 50 percent of appeals result in a decision in favor of the patient.[21]

Document the name of each person you talk to, along with the date and time, and summarize each discussion. Maintain a file of all communications and associated paperwork. Continue to contact the appropriate individuals by phone and/or email, and don't hesitate to pursue your appeal up the chain of command. Some appeals can take several months to resolve. If the insurance company upholds the prior denial and your insurance is through your work, in some instances, you may be allowed to appeal to the company that employs you.

If You Can't Afford Health Insurance or Can't Pay Your Bill

It is a very scary prospect to go without health insurance, particularly if you have medical problems or a family to care for. While the Affordable Care Act (ACA) has options in the state marketplace for those who are unemployed, the plans may still be too expensive for one's budget. In Joe's case, there was a broker or agent designated by the state to help individuals find affordable plans or find cost assistance that may be available. Medicaid eligibility has been expanded in some states, and you will want to see if you qualify. In addition, there may be short-term or temporary health insurance plans as well that offer a limited set of benefits for a specific length of time.

The Emergency Medical Treatment & Labor Act (EMTALA) is a federal law that requires anyone coming to an emergency department to be stabilized and treated, regardless of their insurance status or ability to pay. However, it's important to use the hospital emergency room for true emergencies and not like a doctor's office visit, as you may otherwise still be responsible for the bill. The emergency room is expensive and not meant to provide ongoing care.

Emergency room visits and lengthy hospitalizations can be costly. Even with health insurance, the bill can be overwhelming. If you receive a huge medical bill, there may be several ways to approach this:

- First, is the bill accurate? Ask for an itemized bill with every single charge and review it. Are you being charged for services that were not rendered or were not yours? Hospitals charge for any supplies that were used—even a band-aid. Are the charges reasonable?

- These bills can be hard to understand and can contain a lot of confusing medical jargon. You may want to contact the hospital's billing department for help.

- If you have insurance, have you contacted your insurance company? Tell them you want to request an advocate. If you went out-of-network and it was an emergency, can you appeal the charges?

- Can the bill be negotiated? There are companies that may be able to act on your behalf to negotiate the amount of the bill. They may take a portion of the savings as their fee, but it could be worth it.

- Can you negotiate to have the payments reduced or paid out over time? Can you offer them a smaller settlement to close the matter?

Paying Medical Bills with a Credit Card

According to the Consumer Financial Protection Bureau,[22] 58 percent of debts recorded in collections were for a medical bill. Medical debt is now the most common form of debt on consumer credit reports.

The 2022 KFF survey found approximately one in six adults is paying off credit card bills tied to medical or dental services. Although credit card balances are not recorded as medical debt, the JPMorgan Chase Institute has found the typical cardholder's monthly balance jumped 34 percent after a major medical expense.

Because of the interest rate tied to the credit card, your amount owed can increase even as you pay it down. And depending on how able you are to pay (the amount you pay each month and your timeliness), your credit score can be negatively impacted. In turn, a lower credit rating makes it more difficult and more expensive to purchase and pay for other expenses, like a car or a mortgage, if it does not take you out of the running altogether.

If you have no other viable option (e.g., negotiated payment plan with the provider), finding a credit card that does not accrue interest on carried balances for up to a year is likely the best option for a credit card payment of medical bills.

The No Surprises Act[23]

The No Surprises Act legislation, which took effect in January 2022, provides protections against surprise medical bills from out-of-network healthcare providers, especially when you are faced with an emergency through no fault of your own. The regulations apply to individuals who are covered under a group employer plan, an individual health plan, or an Affordable Care Act (ACA) Marketplace plan.

The act bans:

- Surprise bills for most emergency services, even when the emergency facility or provider is out-of-network and prior approval was not received. Out-of-network care is common in the case of emergencies, and many people are surprised when they receive the follow-up bill from the hospital or healthcare provider.

- Surprise bills from an out-of-network provider as part of a visit to an in-network facility. This applies to non-emergency services, such as anesthesiology, pathology, or radiology provided by an out-of-network provider, as part of your preapproved, in-network procedure.

- Out-of-network balance billing without providing a prior estimate and the patient's consent. Balance billing refers to an out-of-network provider billing the patient for the amount not covered by the insurance plan. (Note: Medicare and Medicaid already prohibit balance billing; this new law now applies to private insurance plans.)

The No Surprises Act also provides patients who have regular Medicare with rights to appeal for coverage of rehabilitation in a nursing home after discharge from the hospital if your stay was designated as observation rather than inpatient.

Healthcare practitioners and facilities should provide an easy-to-understand explanation of your billing protections, including whom to contact if you have concerns or if you believe your protections have been violated. You can still choose to see an out-of-network provider, but you must be told an estimate of the costs ahead of time and give your consent. To avoid balance billing, you'll want to be aware of what you're signing. If you are uninsured or do not use your health insurance for healthcare services, the legislation allows your right to a good-faith estimate of the cost of your care up front, before your visit.

At the time this book is being written, some of the key provisions of the No Surprises Act have been set aside in response to lawsuits by providers. Final decisions will likely be determined by the Department of Justice. As these laws change, it is important to stay up to date on your rights and to advocate for yourself.

ADDITIONAL COST-SAVING IDEAS

- The ACA mandates that all nonprofit hospitals provide financial assistance to patients who need it. Be sure to explore what support is available relative to hospital bills if you meet the eligibility criteria.

- Recognize that this unfortunate situation is faced by many, and you are not alone. Do not let shame, embarrassment, or pride stop you from seeking and accepting help. Waiting will only compound the problem and put you in a more precarious situation.

- Whenever your financial status will allow, set aside and contribute as much as you can afford to an emergency fund.

- Take the time to become financially literate.

- If you have not already, do everything within your control regarding your lifestyle to optimize your health and well-being at every opportunity. Make taking care of yourself a priority. It is an investment in you that will not only make you feel better—mind, body, and spirit—but will help reduce the risk of finding your financial status in peril due to medical conditions that are potentially preventable or at least within a significant degree of your control to manage effectively.

Healthcare in the U.S. is expensive and, despite significant progress attributable to the Affordable Care Act, as well as expansion of the Medicaid program in several states, there are many people who are still uninsured or underinsured. If you are without coverage or have insurance but are hit with a huge medical expense, you will want to investigate your employer, local community, and government resources to help minimize the impact on your financial health.

SO, WHAT CAN YOU DO NOW?

- One of the top reasons for personal bankruptcy in the U.S. is medical bills; that's why health insurance is critical.

- Take the time to educate yourself about your insurance options to determine the best fit for your needs, and be sure to sign up within the enrollment period.

- If you can get insurance through an employer, it may be cheaper than buying it on the open market. If not, see if you qualify for Medicaid, the Affordable Care Act (ACA), or any local funding sources.

- Do an analysis each year, as both health plans and your healthcare needs can change from year to year.

- Stay abreast of changing healthcare-related laws and plan provisions, as they may help provide additional benefits for you and your family.

- If available, take advantage of healthcare savings account features (FSA, HRA/HSA) to help cover your medical expenses, as well as any health-related programs/resources your employer may offer, such as case management, Employee Assistance Program (EAP), or flu clinics.

- If you don't understand the charges on a medical bill or why an insurance claim was denied, be persistent in resolving the issue and do not hesitate to seek help.

CHAPTER 12

Preparing for the End of Life

*We cannot change the outcome,
but we can affect the journey.*

ANN RICHARDSON

NANCY'S STORY ABOUT DEVA

Nancy resided in Maryland, and her 103-year-old mother, Deva, was in Missouri. Deva had lived on a farm for most of her life, was healthy, and rarely visited a doctor. When she was fifty-three years old, Deva's husband died, and she stayed on to manage the farm herself until age eighty-one. Then, after visiting several communities, Deva purchased a house in a fifty-five-and-older continuing care retirement community (CCRC) in Kansas City, so as she aged, she could move into an on-site, assisted-living facility or the nursing center, if needed. During Deva's first year in the house, Nancy's older sister, Elaine, who lived in the same city, moved in with her. Deva enjoyed her new community, became great friends with her neighbors, and participated in various social and volunteer activities.

Deva never wanted to put unnecessary burdens on her children. In her early eighties, with her mind still sharp, she took care of the necessary end-of-life preparations. Working with an attorney, Deva prepared her healthcare advance directive, assigned Elaine as durable power of attorney, updated her will, and purchased long-term care insurance. For many years she remained in good health. She needed medicines for mild glaucoma, bladder urgency, and to control GERD (gastroesophageal reflux disease) caused by a large hiatal hernia she'd had for many years.

In her late nineties, however, Deva began exhibiting short-term memory loss and cognitive decline. This was the beginning of a dementia that altered her life. Elaine, now retired, took over managing her affairs and finances. In May of Deva's 103rd year, she developed a heart condition, atrial fibrillation (Afib), and began taking medication to regulate it. Increasingly frail, Deva now needed assistance with most of the activities of daily living and used a walker to move safely around the house.

As her mother's dementia and weakness progressed, Nancy began traveling to Missouri four or five days every month to help with her care and give her sister a much-needed break. In October of that same year, Elaine broke her arm and had to have surgery. Nancy immediately flew to Missouri and stayed for three weeks to care for both.

Deva had been receiving her primary healthcare at a hospital outpatient senior clinic. In July, the clinic changed from offering full-time primary care services to providing consultation services two days per month. Deva lost her excellent primary care practitioner, who moved to a position in the hospital. After Elaine broke her arm, Nancy drove her mother to a previously scheduled follow-up exam with one of the clinic's consulting geriatric nurse practitioners who had seen Deva once before. The exam went well, and no changes in Deva's care were needed. Knowing that this nurse practitioner also worked in a long-term care facility, Nancy asked to talk to him privately. She wanted to know what to expect as her mother's health continued to deteriorate. He told her a stroke, heart attack, or internal bleeding from a fall would likely end her mother's life. He recommended the family be aware of any spike in Deva's blood pressure, an irregular heartbeat, or shortness of breath, and call 911 if any of those things occurred.

A few days later, in the early hours of the night, Deva experienced a rapidly variable heart rate, very high blood pressure, and shortness of breath. Elaine called 911. When the EMTs (emergency medical technicians) arrived, they said Deva needed to be taken to the ER. The head of the team asked to see Deva's healthcare directive, or living will. In the stress of the moment, Elaine and Nancy could only find an online copy of it, and Elaine's printer was not working. Nancy told him her mother had a DNR (Do Not Resuscitate) order and asked, "Can we show it to you online?"

"No," the EMT said. "I must have a copy of it in my hand and take it with me to the hospital. If anything should happen, I will have to resuscitate her." Nancy followed the ambulance to the hospital. After the ER doctor's exam and a chest x-ray, Nancy was told that in addition to the presenting issues, her mother also had a mild case of pneumonia. Deva was hospitalized to treat the pneumonia and to find a better way to control her Afib and high blood pressure. She was placed in a private room.

In the hospital that day, Deva's dementia and confusion were more pronounced. "I don't know why I'm here," she insisted. "I feel okay and want to go home." Nancy stayed by her mother's side to comfort her, interact with the multiple healthcare providers, and explain what was happening. The only thing Deva could understand was that she had pneumonia and needed to recover. At around 11:00 p.m., the night nurse suggested Nancy go home and rest since she had been up for over twenty-one hours. Although reluctant to leave, Nancy knew she needed to be alert and able to function the next day. Elaine, just a few days post-surgery, would not be able to make trips to the hospital.

At 8:30 a.m. the next morning, Nancy arrived back at the hospital and was informed of her mother's terrible night. Deva had been confused, agitated, and repeatedly tried to get out of bed. She had not slept at all. Her cold, untouched breakfast was sitting on the rolling cart across the room. Nancy knew she needed to find a way to ease her mother's anxiety and make this hospitalization less stressful.

Nancy noticed that the "call button" was on the side table out of her mother's reach. She wrapped the cord around the bed rails and began instructing her mother on its use. It took several training sessions for her mother to understand and remember how to use it.

At mealtime, Nancy placed the rolling food cart across Deva's bed. She could see that even with the bed in a sitting position her petite mother was struggling to reach the food. Deva was capable of feeding herself, so Nancy removed the rolling tray cart, placed a bed pillow on her mother's lap, covered it with a towel, and put the plate on top. This allowed her to easily reach the food.

Deva would get worried if Nancy left the room for more than five minutes, so when Nancy went to the cafeteria for lunch, she left a note saying, "Nancy has gone to lunch. Will be back at 1:30." Deva held on to the piece of paper and watched the clock opposite her bed until Nancy returned. Armed with this knowledge, Deva was able to stay calm. Every time Nancy had to leave, even at night, she left a note about where she would be and what time she would return. Nancy explained the purpose and importance of this note to the hospital staff. Unfortunately, the next afternoon when Nancy had to take Elaine to get her stitches removed, she returned to find her mother very upset and agitated by her absence. Someone had moved the note to the windowsill, and Deva could not remember where Nancy was and even if she would be back.

At bedtime the second night, Nancy turned the lights low, sat by her mother's side, held her hand, stroked her forehead, and talked quietly to her. When Deva drifted off to sleep, Nancy tucked a note into the covers and left without waking her. She spoke to the night staff to inform them her mother was sleeping and asked that she not be disturbed if possible. By this time, the hospital had added a bed alarm so they would be alerted if her mother tried to get out of bed. Also, the addition of an external catheter meant that Deva would not be disturbed by needing to go to the toilet. She was able to sleep some that evening but never was able to get a full night's sleep at the hospital. Her anxiety and confusion worsened at night in such unfamiliar surroundings.

Due to her age, Deva was not a candidate for pacemaker surgery. Her cardiologist explained that she needed stronger medicine to regulate her heartbeat. It had to be built up gradually over about four to five weeks to reach an effective dose, administered intravenously. When she had recovered sufficiently from the pneumonia and could take the meds orally, she could be discharged. However, until the dosage reached an effective level, she would still be at risk for an Afib flareup. In the early evening of the fifth day, Deva was released. She was happy to leave the hospital for the comforts of home.

Looking ahead, Nancy knew she would soon need to return to Maryland. Elaine was not yet able to drive and needed several weeks of physical therapy. While their mother was still in the hospital, they decided it was time to hire a healthcare aide to assist with Deva's care at home. They chose to work with Senior Helpers, since it was a well-respected provider in the retirement community. Nancy called and found that this organization already had a working relationship with Deva's long-term care insurance company. After a period of sixty days, Deva's policy would pay for the daily cost of the in-home aide.

Senior Helpers was able to cover the first few days of Nancy's absence with temporary aides until a permanent person was available. The permanent aide, compassionate and experienced, quickly became indispensable.

Other services and changes helped further address Deva's needs and allow her to remain in her home, where she was most comfortable. Occupational and physical therapy services, covered by Medicare, were provided at home after a three-day hospitalization. Elaine ordered a hospital bed that allowed her mother's head to be slightly raised so she could breathe more comfortably. The house was already equipped with an alert system and had handrails both beside and opposite the toilet in Deva's bathroom. An additional handrail by Deva's bed was installed to help prevent falls when she got up to go into the bathroom at night. The home healthcare aide led Deva through a set of seated and standing exercises to preserve her strength and range of motion. Nancy and Elaine placed pictures of the family on the wall in front of Deva's bedroom chair to help remind her of home.

Deva's modesty was a barrier to having the healthcare aide assist her with showering. Elaine provided a loose, sleeveless, big-necked, terry cloth beach cover-up, and told her mother it was a "shower dress." Deva would sit in the seat in the walk-in shower and the aide could bathe her under the dress. She was comfortable with that arrangement.

Deva's initial hospitalization was followed by three more calls to 911 over the next two months. On two of those occasions, Deva was able to be treated in the ER and released. One episode did require hospitalization for four days. After their first experience with the EMTs, Nancy and Elaine had put a copy of Deva's living will and the DNR order, along with a list of her physicians and medications, in a container on a shelf in the refrigerator. It was always within reach.

At the time of the second hospitalization, in November, Nancy was in Maryland and not able to get there until the day after Deva was discharged. Elaine had recovered enough to be with her mother during those four days but was not yet driving. Through Lyft and friends, she was able to get to and from the hospital.

Nighttime continued to be difficult, as Deva would get scared and confused and have trouble sleeping. Her daughters asked Senior Helpers to provide a nighttime home health aide to spend a couple of nights in the hospital attending to their mother. It did not help. Deva did not know this aide and was confused by her presence. The lack of sleep, increased anxiety, and even some episodes of delusions were of increasing concern and made it harder for Deva to recover. This pattern had begun to happen at home as well. Deva was suffering from "sundown syndrome," common among individuals with dementia. The day Deva was dismissed, Elaine consulted with the attending hospitalist about treatment for these nighttime difficulties. He wrote a prescription for olanzapine, an antipsychotic drug, and explained it was being used for this purpose in Europe. The cardiologist added a prescription for a diuretic to help treat Deva's edema in her feet and ankles caused by poor circulation. The number of daily medicines was growing.

The next day Nancy arrived to help with Deva's care, particularly at night so Elaine could sleep. When they read the insert that came with the olanzapine, they discovered the drug had potentially lethal side effects in elderly patients. They decided not to risk giving it to her.

It was difficult for the family to go through this series of crises without a primary care physician to call who was knowledgeable about Deva's case and health history. Their mother's pulmonologist recommended an internist he knew as a primary care doctor for Deva. They called for an appointment and took their mother to see him. To treat the sundowning, he prescribed an anti-anxiety medication that proved only somewhat effective.

Over time, it became clear that the new internist was not as experienced with the care of the advanced elderly as they had hoped. He was also curt and a bit intimidating in the exam room. The family decided they needed someone who specialized in geriatric care and who was receptive to their questions and concerns.

They knew it was important to have someone who would coordinate with their mother's cardiologist and pulmonologist. They also wanted a comprehensive review of her medications. Should she continue with all the drugs? Should the dosages be adjusted? Was there any concern about adverse interaction among the medicines?

Nancy also researched palliative care resources in the local area. Would someone be able to come to the home? Would this be covered by Medicare or by long-term care insurance? Was this service needed at this point? They agreed to have an in-home educational session with a representative from the palliative care organization to learn more about it. She asked Elaine several questions then called back the next day to say that Deva was not eligible to receive palliative care since she was still leaving the house for physician appointments and other short trips.

In the end, they chose to engage a physician group specializing in geriatrics that was affiliated with Deva's senior community. A geriatric nurse practitioner and a registered nurse were on-site. Supervision was provided by a geriatric specialist physician. The nurse practitioner was able to provide exams and follow-up care right in Deva's home. It was even possible for her to bring diagnostic equipment into the house if an EKG (electrocardiogram) or x-rays were needed. The RN shared her cell phone number and was easily reachable during the day if the family had questions. A nighttime RN was on call if they needed to consult with someone when the office was closed.

Deva's heart condition and health gradually improved. In December, she was able to dress up and celebrate her 104th birthday with her family at a restaurant. Deva was a big hit at the restaurant, with staff and other customers coming over to speak with her. Afterward they drove her though a large holiday light display in a local park. She was delighted by the entire evening.

Unfortunately, Deva's bedtime anxiety and inability to sleep through the night continued. The geriatric nurse practitioner told Nancy and Elaine that their physician group included a geriatric neurologist who specialized in dementia and would see their mother. Nancy made the appointment and went with Elaine and Deva to see the neurologist at her office. This warm and compassionate doctor gave Deva a thorough cognitive and physical evaluation, reviewed all her medications, and answered all their questions. She spent two-and-a-half hours with the family. She told them Deva likely had either cardiovascular dementia or Alzheimer's (or a mixture). She prescribed a different anti-anxiety drug and added an antidepressant. This combination, built up over time, was effective in reducing Deva's nighttime confusion and allowed her to get to sleep without fears and protests.

Due to the dementia, there was little Deva could do, and she became bored. She was no longer able to follow the plot of a TV show, movie, or book. She liked being useful, so Elaine gave her little jobs to do around the house, like folding laundry or grocery bags and arranging clean silverware into a cutlery tray. She enjoyed watching YouTube videos of "The Lawrence Welk Show" and didn't care if she had already seen them. An adviser at the local chapter of the Alzheimer's Association provided other ideas for activities, such as asking her to put a deck of cards into numerical order or sorting mixed colored cards or file folders into categories by color. Previously Deva had enjoyed adult coloring books but could no longer figure out what color to put where. Nancy sent her a "color-by-number" coloring book, and she was able to color again. She loved birds and enjoyed watching them at a bird feeder outside the window by her chair in the living room.

The coronavirus pandemic hit in the spring of 2020. Just days after Nancy's mid-March visit, the executive director of the senior community announced no outside people would be allowed in, other than healthcare workers. Nancy stayed in touch with phone calls, emails, and texts. The healthcare aide continued to visit and wore a mask while she was there. Elaine lined up a close friend on their block to call in case of any future emergencies.

Because Elaine had the responsibility of day-to-day care, Nancy volunteered to provide remote assistance with some of her mother's paperwork and logistics. She was able to handle arrangements and record keeping with the home healthcare agency, fill out various forms, make some appointments, and be the primary contact for the long-term care insurance company.

During the COVID-19 outbreak, the management of the community began periodic testing of every resident and staff member and implemented specific safety, cleanliness, and social distancing measures. They set up an isolation ward with dedicated staff in a separate wing of the nursing center to treat any residents who tested positive for the virus. Over time, some assisted-living and nursing home residents and staff contracted the disease. However, none of the residents in the apartments or independent homes tested positive for the virus. Elaine and Deva stayed at home and had groceries and other necessities delivered.

Three months after celebrating her 105th birthday, Deva's health declined further, and the family sought home hospice services for assistance. Finally, with all of them fully vaccinated, Nancy made it back to her mother's side. Deva passed peacefully in her own home one week later.

Nancy feels gratified she was able to spend time those months with her mother and sister before COVID-19 put a stop to all visits for a year. Although it was always difficult to leave, she knew Deva was receiving good care. Despite the dementia, Nancy and Elaine had some wonderful moments with their mother and knew they were a comfort to her during the remaining days of her life.

LESSONS LEARNED

- Managing the care of a patient at the end of life requires a great deal of time and attention. Knowing what to expect and how to handle debilitating and terminal medical conditions can be a challenging job.

- To address the needs of any patient, finding the right clinician is key. In the case of an aging parent, finding a geriatric specialist can be helpful. And support from a home health aide can make all the difference if you can afford one, making long-term care insurance even more beneficial.

- Necessary adjustments to the home environment might be necessary to ensure safety and comfort.

- Being prepared in advance with the proper documents—a living will and DNR order, for example—can ensure that your wishes or those of a loved one are honored.

- Coordinating the care of someone at the end of life, especially when several medications and specialists are involved, is key to comfort and well-being. Additional resources, such as palliative care and hospice, can be especially helpful during this time and may offer help that might not otherwise be affordable.

WHAT YOU NEED TO KNOW

In 2021, there were roughly fifty-two million people, or 16.5 percent of the population, over the age of sixty-five in the United States.[1] By 2030, seniors will outnumber children.[2] Along with this aging population come many health challenges with chronic illnesses, such as heart disease, diabetes, obesity, and dementia, as well as disabilities from frailty and underlying medical conditions. The National Health and Aging Trends Study[3] shows that just over 20 percent of adults aged sixty-five to sixty-nine have poor capacity (physical limitations, poor vision, poor hearing, or probable dementia), while more than 80 percent have poor capacity by age ninety. Because these conditions can extend over a period of several years, the emotional and financial burden on caregivers and the healthcare system can be enormous.

Racial, ethnic, sex, and socioeconomic health disparities exist among the elderly as well and are significant determinants in the amount and quality of healthcare they receive. Rural areas are reported to have the highest concentrations of older people and are aging faster than urban areas.[4] Like their younger counterparts, older people living in rural locations often have access to fewer healthcare services and face longer travel times to obtain care.

Moreover, the pool of traditional family caregivers for older Americans is shrinking. Baby boomers experienced more divorce and had fewer children than previous generations. Although multigenerational living is more common in certain cultures and among those who have recently immigrated to the U.S., family members are more geographically dispersed. Even if they do have adult children, seniors may find these children are ill prepared, unable, or unwilling to take on the care of an aging parent. Some may also have children who are struggling to meet their own day-to-day needs and often carry significant debt, perhaps related to educational loans. Working full time, managing a household, and raising their own children may leave little time to

DROP IN LIFE EXPECTANCY[5]

- In 2022, COVID-19 was one of the major causes of death in the U.S.

- According to the CDC (Centers for Disease Control and Prevention), during the course of the pandemic, overall life expectancy in the U.S. fell in both 2020 and 2021. In 2019, life expectancy was 78 years, 10 months. At the end of 2021, it was 76 years, 1 month.

- Life expectancy for Native Americans, whose level in 2021 (at age 65) was much lower than the average, dropped by 6.5 years between 2019 and 2021.

- Aside from COVID-19, other factors contributing to the decline included suicide and opioid overdoses.

provide regular, much less round-the-clock, care for an aging parent, especially one with chronic conditions. This puts an additional demand on nursing homes, assisted-living facilities, and home healthcare and hospice services, all of which are expensive and well beyond the financial reach of much of the population. Staffing shortages resulting from the COVID-19 pandemic have made a bad situation even worse.

Nancy and Elaine were fortunate. Until the last couple of years, their mother had been healthy most of her life. She had lived a frugal lifestyle that allowed her to pay for both health and long-term care insurance and to be financially independent. She also had the benefit of two children who were both willing and able to share caregiving responsibilities. While other families may not be so fortunate, there are many lessons from their experience.

Be Prepared

The first step is to proactively plan and prepare. Before her health and mental state began to deteriorate, their mother worked with an attorney to create an advance directive, or living will, a document designed to guide her loved ones regarding her end-of-life wishes in the event she would be unable to make those decisions in the future. It addressed such questions as:

- If you are in a coma or vegetative state and would have a very poor quality of life, would you want doctors to use aggressive measures to prolong your life (e.g., breathing machines, resuscitation, dialysis, IV nutrition, etc.)?

- Whom do you authorize to make healthcare-related decisions on your behalf?

- Do you want to donate any organ, tissue, or body part upon your death?

- What is most important for how you want to spend your last days (e.g., no pain, family members present, etc.)?

These are topics that are ideally discussed with your loved ones long before such a document comes into play. Many senior communities, doctors, and hospitals ask for the advance directive to have in their records, but barely one-third of seniors have developed one.

For those seniors with traditional Medicare, consider obtaining a "medigap" insurance policy or supplemental plan, which will help pay for services and expenses not covered by Medicare. Long-term care insurance can also be an economic lifesaver if purchased early, when a person is healthy enough to obtain an affordable, quality policy. (Note: Purchasing long-term care insurance in one's twenties is not too soon!) Also, disability insurance is a good option, if possible, to cover living expenses and medical care at any age, in the event of disability by a severe accident or debilitating disease.

Take Precautions

We've discussed in earlier chapters the importance and positive impact of preventive care and having a support network and a sense of both purpose and community. The value of each of these factors only increases as we age. There are several preventive measures that can be taken, budget permitting, that might include the following:

1. Adjust the home environment to avoid falls and injury.
    - Install grab bars in the shower and tub, and add a

shower bench if room allows. Use bath/shower mats with strong gripping action.
- Install a more elevated seat for the commode and grab bars beside the toilet.
- Secure handrails by the stairs.
- Remove throw rugs and keep the floor clear to avoid trip-and-fall risks.
- Buy kitchen tools to help with opening jars and cans.
- Place items in easy-to-reach places in the kitchen.
- Buy plug-in night lights to make it easy to see the way to the bathroom.
- Purchase a bed that allows for elevation of the head and legs.
- If mobility is limited or climbing the stairs is a problem, research options such as motorized chair lifts and/or consider living on the first floor. If wheelchair-bound, consider building a ramp to enter the house.

2. Consider subscribing to a medical alert service.

3. Address any vision and hearing impairments with glasses, hearing aids, cataract surgery, etc. Use accessibility features on TVs, computers, and cell phones to adjust the font size and backgrounds.

4. Encourage physical activity to help maintain muscle strength, flexibility, and balance. For example, you might consider a website like Daily Dose PD.

5. Speak up. In a culture that is youth-oriented, it is common for older adults to find themselves "invisible" in the healthcare system. For example, even though a loved one

may have full cognitive abilities, a physician may tend to direct all questions to you, even with the patient sitting right beside you. And when speaking to an older individual, conversations may be paternal in nature, with the person being treated like a helpless child.

6. Attach a copy of any DNR (Do Not Resuscitate) orders and power of attorney documentation in an envelope on the outside door of the refrigerator. Most EMTs are trained to look there first.

7. Keep an updated list of medications, including any supplements and OTC (over-the-counter) items, including the dosage, frequency, and time taken. The list should be readily available for caregivers, hospice personnel, EMTs, inpatient staff, and office visits.

Coordinate Care

Depending on their health conditions, many older adults often see several different specialists. As with all patients, it is important for seniors to have a primary care practitioner who knows them and their medical history and can coordinate care among different specialists. Nancy and Elaine realized the lack of a trusted PCP was a problem for their mother and found a geriatric specialty group to treat her. They made a list of all her physicians and medications to bring to appointments with all involved in her care. They also put a list of the physicians and medications, along with the advance directive, in an easily accessible place in case of an emergency.

According to the American Academy of Family Physicians (AAFP), the average elderly patient is taking more than five prescription medications; the average nursing home patient is taking seven medications. Keeping track of these medications, filling and refilling prescriptions, monitoring side effects or drug interactions, and remembering to take them as prescribed can be challenging, especially for those with a cognitive disability. Often, a multi-drug regimen itself can negatively impact cognition and make adherence even more challenging.

It is helpful to use the same pharmacy to keep track of all medications and to provide any notifications of potential problems. Most pharmacies now provide an auto-refill service, and many offer home delivery to avoid gaps in medication adherence. Some insurers have mail-order services, which mean fewer trips to the pharmacy and often result in lower out-of-pocket costs. Some physician groups or health systems may have embedded pharmacists who review medication regimens to optimize dosing, monitor side effects, and reduce the likelihood of drug-drug interactions. Many health insurers make pharmacists available to members, may be able to help with accessing discount programs from manufacturers, and may coordinate specialty medications (usually medications involving home injection). Depending on the health insurance coverage in place or in situations with no insurance or no pharmacy benefit, discount cards like Good Rx can reduce the financial burden of medication, the cost of which continues to rise unabated.

Nancy and Elaine monitored their mother's medications for any adverse reactions or change in condition and proactively contacted the healthcare provider with their concerns. They kept track of whether their mother took her medications at the right time and refilled the prescriptions in advance when the supply was running low. If the dosage or medication changed, they informed the primary care practitioner of any adjustments.

Be an Advocate

After the move to the continuing care community, at least one of the daughters was able to accompany their mother to all physician visits and to be present during any hospitalizations. They acted as her advocate for all aspects of her care. Whether it was the food tray, the call button, or Deva's nighttime anxiety, they addressed these issues with the nurses and physicians on her behalf. With staff having so many patients to treat, it is often difficult for nurses and doctors to have an in-depth understanding of each patient's needs, so it's critical for family members and caregivers to speak up when there's an issue.

The choice of care settings for seniors can be a difficult decision. Depending on the extent of care required, one's financial means, and the availability of options where one lives, caregivers may have some hard decisions to make. Can mom or dad live independently and "age in place"? Can the home be set up to accommodate a disability or limited mobility? Can a home healthcare aide assist with some daily activities—dressing, toileting, bathing, or cooking? Are there funds (personal, long-term care insurance, federal/state/local programs) available for these options?

Is there a senior facility that provides safety and security for its residents, along with a customized health and well-being program? Are seniors able to engage in activities so they can interact with others, or are they just left alone to sit and watch TV from one meal to the next?

The Centers for Medicare and Medicaid provide information on hospitals and nursing homes that allows you to compare facilities on a number of quality and cost measures. Recent hurricanes like Katrina and Ian led to devastating flooding where older adults were the most vulnerable. And during the coronavirus pandemic, residents of nursing homes, assisted-living facilities, and veterans' homes were especially hit hard. Without the ability to have visitors, many residents were unable to have family members check on them; they suffered greatly from fear, isolation, and loneliness, and often died alone. Nancy and Elaine were fortunate their senior community acted quickly when the COVID-19 crisis began.

Seek Additional Resources

Palliative care

If caring for someone with a serious illness, an important resource for caregivers is the palliative care team. Palliative care specialists work in partnership with the doctor to provide additional support for a patient who may be in severe pain or stress from cancer, heart disease, Alzheimer's, Parkinson's, and many other conditions. The goal of palliative care is to provide the best possible quality of life for the patient, and it is usually covered by most insurance plans, including Medicare and Medicaid. With a focus on relieving pain and other symptoms of a serious, life-threatening condition, palliative care can also include emotional, spiritual, and practical support. It can help patients and the family through the stresses of multiple hospitalizations and debilitating side effects of ongoing treatment. Caregivers will want to ask the doctor or nurse in the hospital or other healthcare facility to see a palliative care specialist when needed.

PALLIATIVE CARE FACTS[6]

- The Center to Advance Palliative Care (CAPC) and the National Palliative Care Research Center (NPCRC) found that, as of 2019, the availability of palliative care was impacted by geographic locale. For example, availability was greater in the Northeast than in the South. And 90 percent of hospitals with palliative care are in urban areas.
- Nonprofit hospitals are more likely to provide palliative care services than their for-profit counterparts.
- Palliative care services are more likely to be available in hospitals with 300 or more beds than in smaller ones.

Hospice care

Although hospice care may involve palliative care, they are not the same thing. Hospice care can provide welcome support if a patient is in the final phase of a terminal illness, no longer receiving curative treatment or the patient and family have declined further treatment, and a doctor certifies life expectancy is six months or less. The goal of hospice care is to help patients live as comfortably and free of pain as possible, while maintaining a patient's dignity, in their remaining days. Depending on the patient's status, hospice services may be delivered in the home, in a nursing home, in an inpatient setting, or at a facility specifically designated for hospice.

When you agree to hospice care, you will receive services by professionals trained to deal with end-of-life issues. With limited physical activity, declining mental alertness, or the body in a weakened state, a patient's ability to take care of activities of daily living (ADLs)—like personal hygiene, eating, and dressing—as well as mobility and maintaining continence can become severely diminished. Depending on your hospice benefit, it may cover such services as a home health aide, DME (durable medical equipment), and grief counseling for your family and other loved ones. In addition to pain management, other

---

WHO RECEIVES HOSPICE CARE?[7]

A 2021 report by the National Hospice and Palliative Care Organization (NHPCO) indicated that in 2019:

- Of Medicare beneficiaries who died, 51.9 percent received one or more days of hospice services.
- More patients who identified as women utilized hospice services than those who identified as men.
- The greatest percentage of Medicare patients who used hospice were age eighty-five or older.
- There were differences in utilization of hospice by race/ethnicity, in this descending order: White > Hispanic/Latino > Black > Asian > Indigenous Peoples.
- The top five diagnoses for which hospice services were utilized were Alzheimer's, heart disease, stroke, cancer, and lung disease.
- The average length of stay for 50 percent of patients was eighteen days or less.

services may include antibiotics for infections that are easily treated and respite care.

In addition to the expertise and support available, hospice can lighten another complicated and common burden on caregivers. Although a hospice nurse does not manage medication, they may help by physically allocating a patient's pills to a pillbox system, thereby reducing confusion, increasing adherence, and assuring no gaps in refill prescriptions. Out-of-pocket costs may also be reduced significantly depending on the medication regimen and the pharmacy coverage that may be available.

Coverage for hospice services can vary depending on the type of insurance you have and your ability to pay out of pocket. So, it is important to obtain the details of what your insurance plan includes and the specific services covered. If the patient is covered through Medicare, there is no charge to the patient.

It is common for people to believe hospice only applies to people with cancer. However, other examples include patients with end-stage heart failure or end-stage COPD (chronic obstructive pulmonary disease). Studies have shown that, unfortunately, a request for hospice is frequently long delayed, often until the last few weeks or days of a patient's life. Healthcare providers are often not trained in having difficult conversations about the end of life and may find it particularly uncomfortable. Some patients and their families find it difficult to accept that the final stage of illness has been reached. However, once they start to experience the many benefits of this type of compassionate care, many have wished they had availed themselves of the services sooner. Hospice can be a wonderful resource for caregivers, as it allows the patient and the family to focus on their last days together, get their affairs in order, and say their goodbyes.

Taking care of aging parents with failing physical and/or mental health, or of someone with a terminal illness, can often be a full-time job for family members or other caregivers. Ensuring they have the right level of care in a safe environment is critical. Obtaining specialized resources like geriatric and/or end-of-life care is key. Of utmost importance, however, is to engage in end-of-life conversations early and to document a person's wishes. Having a plan, and adjusting it when health conditions change, can go a long way to making optimal decisions under less pressure at a very difficult time.

Although this chapter has focused on end-of-life situations for those in an elderly demographic, much of what has been covered is applicable across a wide range of ages. The fundamentals are universal, and many of the options apply regardless of age.

SO, WHAT CAN YOU DO NOW?

- The only guarantee in life is death. Most people are uncomfortable and/or hesitant to think about their mortality because of fear of the unknown. However, taking steps early to organize your affairs and plan for the inevitable often provides a sense of control as well as comfort, knowing you have made the necessary preparations for the future.

- Your physical and mental health needs will likely change in a variety of ways as you grow older. Be proactive and make any necessary adjustments to accommodate an evolving health status so you can live as independently as possible and optimize your quality of life.

- If available, consider a consultation by a geriatrician.

- Get clarity about your wishes or those of your loved one in enough detail to complete documents like a living will, power of attorney, and advance directives.

- Make a file (and keep it up to date) that includes information about bank accounts, safe deposit boxes, insurance policies, 401(k) and other retirement accounts, beneficiaries, Social Security, veteran benefits, etc., for easy access.

- Declutter and purge on a regular basis to make life as easy as possible for anyone who will be involved in closing out your affairs.

- Make arrangements for your funeral/memorial service, and prepay for services if you can afford to do so.

Epilogue

*The best preparation for tomorrow
is doing your best today.*
                                    H. JACKSON BROWN JR.

As we conclude work on our book, we've entered the third year of the pandemic, and many of us are experiencing COVID-19 exhaustion. While some are returning to the office, many in-person events and social activities have resumed, and masking requirements have relaxed, some businesses are still struggling to stay afloat. People continue to be concerned about the long-term effects of the virus and what future variants may emerge. And for those who are immunocompromised, life and the workplace have become even more complicated.

Given the number of U.S. hospitalizations and a death toll surpassing one million, healthcare workers have experienced a high degree of stress, fatigue, and a feeling of being overworked and unappreciated. This has led to significant staffing shortages in hospitals and healthcare facilities and a wave of retirements. The rates of infection, hospitalizations, and death in certain populations, along with inequitable access to therapeutic treatment, have shone a bright light on many long-standing health disparities. Our mental and emotional health, particularly that of our children, has been impacted significantly. Our world has changed, and a different "normal" will exist as the pandemic becomes less front and center and moves to endemic status.

At the same time, the pandemic has triggered remarkable and rapid advances in medical knowledge, with vaccines and treatments developed in record time. We've seen significant innovations in technology and the delivery of care. Global collaboration has been enhanced as COVID-19 has shown the degree to which the world is now connected, and the impact that one part of the globe can have on all our lives.

Considering the current environment, the messages of this book are even more important now. We must ask questions, seek credible scientific information, consider options, and do our best to optimize our health. The benefits of living a healthy lifestyle and taking the necessary preventive actions have been fully demonstrated. And, given a healthcare system that is still trying to adapt and manage through a highly volatile environment, it is even more critical to advocate for yourself and your loved ones, and to navigate the healthcare system with greater knowledge, confidence, and a willingness to ask for what you need and deserve.

A Master Class

COVID-19 has provided a real-world master class in prevention, self-advocacy, and navigation of the healthcare system.

COVID-19 was the condition selected as an example because all of us have been affected in one way or another by the pandemic. We have all had to learn about the impact on our health and well-being in a short amount of time, and the lessons learned reinforce the messages conveyed in this book. With the pandemic as context, here's a recap of the key lessons from each chapter.

Taking Charge of Your Health

COVID-19 is a novel coronavirus, which means it is new and not something we have experienced before. Therefore, we have had to continually learn and remain open to changing guidance over time as new information has become available. The pandemic has made clear the importance of being willing to ask questions and persist in getting the care you need. When things are uncertain, advocacy for yourself or loved ones becomes paramount.

Embracing a Healthier Lifestyle

Those with underlying medical conditions—such as obesity, diabetes, COPD (chronic obstructive pulmonary disease), heart disease, and cancer—have been at increased risk for hospitalization and death if they developed a COVID-19 infection. Many of these conditions are lifestyle-related, and a healthy lifestyle is important to their management. In addition, the transmissibility of the virus impacted our ability and willingness to obtain preventive care. The rate of cancer screenings, such as mammograms and colonoscopies, plummeted and resulted in a lost chance of early detection for some. Thus, the pandemic has highlighted the critical importance of preventive care and maintaining a healthy lifestyle. Both can reduce the risk of a chronic condition or the development of cancer and can minimize the risk of becoming immunocompromised and more vulnerable as a result.

Choosing the Type of Doctor You Need

Determining the type of doctor you need, or if a second opinion would be beneficial, can be confusing under the best of circumstances. COVID-19 is a virus capable of impacting all the body's organs and systems, including the lungs, heart, brain, and immune system. For those suffering from long COVID, a variety of specialists have been needed at any given time over the course of the illness.

Knowing the type of physician and the focus of each of the specialties is important information to understand. It means you are in a better position to ask for the type of expertise needed in your situation and to optimize the likelihood of getting both an accurate diagnosis and a treatment regimen that will address your condition as soon as possible.

Partnering with Your Doctor

COVID-19 has demonstrated the importance of having someone in your corner who knows you as a whole person—your personal and family history, your preferences and health beliefs, as well as your current social and economic situation. Having a medical professional whom you trust and with whom you can collaborate is key, particularly with a condition like COVID-19, which is complicated and makes advocacy and navigation much more complex. Collaborating with someone who has your best interests at heart, as well as the medical training to provide guidance, is important to your overall health and well-being in general and even more so in the midst of a pandemic.

Coordinating Care

For those who contract COVID-19 and whose symptoms continue to linger, coordination of care may be critically necessary. Long COVID is a condition in which patients may suffer from a range of symptoms—including fatigue, shortness of breath, body/joint aches, loss of taste/smell, digestive issues, or depression—that may last weeks, months, or even years after the infection. Given the array of the body's organs and systems impacted, a team of healthcare practitioners from a variety of specialty areas may need to work together to develop and implement an effective treatment plan. Without adequate communication and collaboration, a patient could easily receive conflicting or inappropriate treatment, and get confused or frustrated as they try to get well.

Having a Baby

Pregnant women have talked with their doctors about the safety of the vaccine on their baby's health. We've seen that those with COVID-19 infections are more vulnerable to severe complications, hospitalization, and death, and their babies are at greater risk of being born prematurely and having a low birth weight. Having a healthy lifestyle prior to conception and during pregnancy reduces the risk of infection and the potential implications for both mother and baby.

Deciding Where to Go When a Medical Condition Strikes

Your primary care practitioner is a good resource for providing guidance about the best place to go for your health concerns. However, figuring that out has been more difficult during the pandemic, as access to some clinical care settings has been limited. Many have used telehealth or a virtual care option to avoid potential exposure during an in-person office visit. As many emergency rooms have become overwhelmed, patients have made greater use of urgent care centers, as well as lab and imaging facilities. Nurse lines, offered by your local health system or by your employer's benefit plan, have become another resource to help determine if your issue can be handled at home. As seen with COVID-19, our health and well-being can change quickly and dramatically. Being aware of the variety of healthcare settings, along with the services each offers, is important—in advance of when a condition strikes.

Maintaining Your Emotional Health

The pandemic has resulted in global emotional distress and has caused much uncertainty, confusion, and anxiety. Everyone has been impacted. People have mourned the loss of a family member, been haunted by the isolation and hospitalization of a loved one, and agonized about their children who have had to attend school virtually—thus missing out on social interaction with their classmates.

Making a commitment to your emotional health, and valuing it as much as your physical well-being, are investments in living life as fully as possible. Your emotional and physical health are inextricably linked. Some people are naturally able to go with the flow, to accept their emotions without judgment, and to recover from setbacks with relative ease. For everyone else, the good news is that resilience and grit are skills that can be cultivated and will serve you in good stead. There are many coping techniques you can use to support your emotional health. Don't be afraid to try some until you find the ones that are the best fit for you.

Dealing with Mental Illness

Along with emotional distress, the pandemic has also negatively impacted those with addictions and other mental health conditions. With the loss of a normal life and the compounding effects of depression and anxiety, some people have increased their alcohol consumption and drug use. Those with mental health conditions like schizophrenia and bipolar disorder, who have contracted COVID-19, have also become more vulnerable to hospitalization and death. And stressed and fatigued hospital workers, overwhelmed by the influx of cases, have suffered from burnout and the symptoms of PTSD (post-traumatic stress disorder).

Addressing mental health disorders within the U.S. healthcare system can be even more fraught than for medical conditions. Learning about the resources available and understanding one's rights are important to obtaining appropriate treatment and quality care.

Facing Health Disparities

The pandemic has put a spotlight on the far-reaching health disparities within segments of the population, which are baked into the U.S. healthcare system. Sex, age, race/ethnicity, socioeconomic status, gender identity, disability status, and geographic locale have all been on display as sources of difference in the risks of COVID infection, complications, and death, as well as in access to preventive measures and quality care. Communities of color have experienced much higher rates of infection, hospitalization, complications, and death than their white counterparts. Those in rural areas continue to have less access to care due to the dearth of medical professionals and hospital closures prior to the pandemic. In addition, rural populations have suffered from the digital divide due to the lack of adequate broadband coverage, which makes virtual care out of reach for many.

Health inequity can threaten your ability to get the type and quality of care you need, as well as the ability to afford preventive measures. It is critical to advocate for yourself and your loved ones. Having the confidence to ask questions and communicate expectations about your care are important to overcoming inequities you may face within the healthcare system.

Paying for Healthcare

Nationally, the cost of COVID-19 has been enormous. For those patients requiring care in a hospital ICU and on a ventilator, the cost can average well over $100,000, and the costs of outpatient care can be $1,000 or more. Depending on the type of insurance coverage, out-of-pocket costs due to co-pays, coinsurance, and deductibles can be several hundred or even several thousand dollars. And for those without any health insurance coverage, the costs are even greater.

Medical debt is one of the top reasons for personal bankruptcy in the U.S. If you have health insurance, it is important to spend the time to select the best plan for your circumstance given the type of medical expenses you anticipate. Those may change from year to year, so understanding what each option covers is important. Additionally, taking advantage of well-being offerings and case management programs helps ensure you are "getting your money's worth" and can help prevent or minimize the risk of certain conditions. This action could lower the cost of future care.

Preparing for potential possibilities, such as becoming disabled or needing long-term care, can also help defray future costs. Investigating and purchasing those types of coverage at a young age typically means lower premium costs and more affordability. Patients with long COVID have sometimes found themselves in a situation in which they needed one or both types of coverage.

Preparing for the End of Life

COVID-19 has been particularly devastating for patients at high risk of severe complications and death from the virus. For the protection of family members and others, hospitalized patients and those in senior living facilities experienced mandatory visiting restrictions. Many have died with no one by their side except the healthcare heroes who have been providing care. The pandemic has been a reminder of the importance of proactively making our wishes known through an advance directive and the assignment of our healthcare proxies to carry out those wishes, including the use of palliative and/or hospice care during the final days of one's life.

A Final Word

The pandemic has pushed all of us to change and adapt quickly. Now is the time to reboot and focus more than ever on our health and well-being. Taking the necessary action to learn and become better prepared can help reduce the risks and complications of illness and help you obtain the right care, from the right person(s), at the right time, in the right place.

As we bring our book to a close, we hope the messages from those who have shared their stories, along with the lessons learned from our own experiences and expertise, will serve as a guiding light on your health and well-being journey, wherever it may lead.

Acknowledgments

*No one who achieves success does so without
acknowledging the help of others.
The wise ... acknowledge this help with gratitude.*

ALFRED NORTH WHITEHEAD

This book represents the contributions and experiences of many individuals for whom we are truly grateful.

First, we wish to thank the individuals who graciously offered to share their stories, even if they were painful to recall. We have not identified them here by name to protect their anonymity. Their hope in discussing these experiences with the healthcare system was to help others who may face similar situations.

We also appreciate the support and guidance of the Bold Story Press team, including Emily Barrosse, Nedah Rose, and Julianna Scott Fein, who have facilitated the publication of our book.

Charlene: Many thanks to my long-time friends and colleagues who agreed to read the draft of our manuscript and provided input and feedback before submission to the publisher. Several had written books of their own and offered valuable publishing and marketing advice. I am truly grateful for the input and feedback of the following individuals —Nancy Batson, MA, ACC; Ellie Beals (author of *Emergence*); Katharine Giacalone (author of *Oops! I'm the Manager! Getting Past "What Do I Do Now?!" in 5 Easy Steps*); Mary G. Jackson, MEd, MS, LCPC (author of *Presence: Recognizing the Divine in Your Everyday Life*); Mary Kemmer (author of *Intangibles*), Kay Labare, MS, Emily Moise, MA; Diane Sarosi, RN; and Carolyn Weiss, APRN.

I am forever grateful for the many friends and family members who provided care and support during my recovery from brain tumor surgery and throughout the subsequent procedures. During the two weeks after my initial surgery, many friends and family members—too numerous to name—took shifts at my house in case I had another seizure. I especially appreciate the support of my friend Nancy Caplan, who coordinated the two-week schedule of everyone's visit. I also owe much gratitude to my dedicated HR team who sent food and kept everything on track in my absence.

I also want to acknowledge several very special physicians who provided excellent care and ultimately helped me get through my lengthy healthcare experience: Dr. Elliot Aleskow, Dr. Henry Brem, Dr. Paul Manson, and Dr. David Hellmann. I especially appreciate the healing power of zero balancing and Qigong master, Karl Ardo, who encouraged my pursuit of health and wellness coaching.

Most importantly, I want to thank my husband, David, and my children, Michael and Emily, whose love and support have helped me through it all and who continue to be the primary source of joy and happiness in my life.

Colette: Many thanks to my beta readers for their support and frank feedback: Amanda Hopkins Tirrell, MBA, FACHE; Carol Oravec, RN; David Nash, MD, MBA; David Katz, MD, MPH; Jay Fischer, MBA; Jane Ehrman, MEd, CHES, CHT; Mary Doherty, DNP MSN, Ed, BSN, RN; Corinne Fisher, PhD; Saria Saccocio, MD, FAAFP, MHA; Linda Roszak Burton, ACC, BBC, BS; Phyllis Cross, MD; Magda Barini-Garcia, MD MBA; Jenn Strathman, Briana Evans, MBA; Mattie Edwards, EdD; and Tanise I. Edwards, MD.

In addition to the beta readers, I appreciate the input of several colleagues who are published authors and offered lessons learned and promotion and marketing tips they found helpful in the process: David Nash, MD MBA; Ruchin Kansal, MBA; David Fagjenbaum, MD, MBA, MSc, FCPP; Ankit Mahadevia, MD, MBA; and Jill Ebstein, MBA.

I would like to thank those who took a particular interest in my education and training—medical, business, coaching, and health equity. I am grateful for a high-school education at an all-girls school that encouraged my curiosity and thirst for learning and empowered me to speak up, express an opinion, and demonstrate an ability in math and science as great as in the humanities; and a college education that brought lessons in how the world often really operates and led to an interest in economics. Although I had always known I wanted to be a physician, that exposure resulted in the pursuit of both an MD and an MBA, with a goal of having the greatest potential impact in the healthcare arena and making a difference in the world.

I am also thankful for the support that contributed to the confidence to pursue an untraditional career in health care. That pathway has provided a broad spectrum of rich experiences and three powerful lessons: (1) the power of the patient-physician relationship regardless of the role in which I have served, (2) the power of focusing on the patient as a whole person with a life (and loved ones) spent primarily outside of the healthcare system, and (3) the commitment to doing right by the patient/member/consumer. Doing so allows one to look at oneself in the mirror, to sleep well at night, and to bring clarity to decisions in complex and complicated situations. All three mean less stress, more satisfaction, greater trust, and better physical and mental health and well-being outcomes.

Resources

CHAPTER 1

Taking Charge of Your Health

Books
- Mary I. O'Connor, MD, and Kanwal L. Haq, MS, T*aking Care of You: The Empowered Woman's Guide to Better Health*, Rochester, MN: Mayo Clinic Press, 2022.

Articles
- "Be More Engaged in Your Healthcare," Agency for Healthcare Research and Quality (AHRQ), reviewed December 2020, https://www.ahrq.gov/questions/be-engaged.
- Jeff Blyskal and Checkbook Staff, "Take Charge of Your Healthcare," Consumers' Checkbook, updated May 2022, https://www.checkbook.org/national/doctors/articles/Take-Charge-of-Your-Healthcare-7291.
- Patient Engagement HIT newsletter, xtelligent Healthcare Media, https://patientengagementhit.com/.
- "Take Charge of Your Health Care/Take Action," MyHealthfinder, Office of Disease Prevention and Health Promotion (OASH), U.S. Department of Health & Human Services, updated July 15, 2022, https://health.gov/myhealthfinder/doctor-visits/talking-doctor/take-charge-your-health-care#take-action-tab.
- "Self-management: Taking Charge of Your Health," familydoctor.org, American Academy of Family Physicians, updated October 19, 2017, https://familydoctor.org/self-management-taking-charge-of-your-health/.
- Chris Woolston, "Taking Charge of Your Healthcare," *HealthDay*, updated June 27, 2022, https://consumer.healthday.com/encyclopedia/patient-safety-32/safety-and-public-health-news-585/taking-charge-of-your-healthcare-648144.html.

- "Information for Consumers and Patients/Drugs," U.S. Food and Drug Administration (FDA), August 8, 2022, https://www.fda.gov/drugs/resources-you-drugs/information-consumers-and-patients-drugs.
- Tara Parker-Pope, "Need Help in a Hospital? Call a Patient Advocate," *New York Times*, March 18, 2022, https://www.nytimes.com/2022/03/03/well/live/hospital-patient-advocates.html.
- "Surgical Risk Calculator," American College of Surgeons (ACS) National Surgical Quality Improvement Program (NSQIP), November 11, 2021, https://riskcalculator.facs.org/RiskCalculator/.
- Jen Gunter, MD, "Looking for accurate health information online? 6 tips to find it, from a doctor," Ideas.Ted.com, September 9, 2021, https://ideas.ted.com/6-tips-for-finding-accurate-health-info-online-health-research/.

CHAPTER 2

Embracing a Healthier Lifestyle

Books

- Mark Hyman, MD, *Food Fix: How to Save Our Health, Our Economy, Our Communities, and Our Planet—One Bite at a Time*, New York: Little, Brown Spark, 2020.
- Dan Buettner, *The Blue Zones Challenge: A 4-Week Plan for a Longer, Better Life*, Washington, DC: National Geographic, 2021.
- Z. Colette Edwards, MD, MBA. *Be Less Stressed*. Maryland: Ingram Spark, 2016. https://peopletweaker.com/guided-steps-less-stressed/.
- Tom Rath, *Eat Move Sleep: Why Small Changes Make a Big Difference*. Arlington, Virginia: Missionday, LLC, 2013.

Articles

- Katie Stiles, reviewed by Lori Lawrenz, "The Importance of Connection," PsychCentral, Updated November 14, 2021, https://psychcentral.com/lib/the importance-of-connection#tips.
- "Immunization Schedules," Centers for Disease Control and Prevention (CDC), reviewed February 17, 2022, https://www.cdc.gov/vaccines/schedules/.
- "Dietary Guidelines for Americans, 2020–2025, 9th Edition," U.S. Department of Agriculture and U.S. Department of Health and Human Services, December 2020, https://www.dietaryguidelines.gov/resources/consumer-resources.

- "Physical Activity Guidelines for Americans, 2nd Edition," Office of Disease Prevention and Health Promotion (ODPHP), U.S. Department of Health and Human Services, updated August 25, 2021, https://health.gov/our-work/nutrition-physical-activity/physical-activity-guidelines.
- "How Much Sleep Do I Need?" Centers for Disease Control and Prevention (CDC), reviewed September 14, 2022, https://www.cdc.gov/sleep/about_sleep/how_much_sleep.html.
- "Coping with Stress," Centers for Disease Control and Prevention (CDC), reviewed November 30, 2021, https://www.cdc.gov/violenceprevention/about/copingwith-stresstips.html.

Cancer Screening Recommendations/Guidelines:

- "Cancer Screening Guidelines by Age," American Cancer Society, accessed November 19, 2022, https://www.cancer.org/healthy/find-cancer-early/cancer-screening-guidelines/screening-recommendations-by-age.html.
- "Mammography Saves Lives," American College of Radiology (ACR), accessed November 19, 2022, https://www.acr.org/Practice-Management-Quality-Informatics/Practice-Toolkit/Patient-Resources/Mammography-Saves-Lives.
- "Updated Cervical Cancer Screening Guidelines," American College of Obstetricians and Gynecologists (ACOG), accessed November 19, 2022, https://www.acog.org/clinical/clinical-guidance/practice-advisory/articles/2021/04/updated-cervical-cancer-screening-guidelines.
- "Colorectal Cancer Guidelines," Medscape, updated March 7, 2022, https://emedicine.medscape.com/article/2500006-overview
- "Saved By the Scan," American Lung Association, accessed November 19, 2022, https://www.lung.org/lung-health-diseases/lung-disease-lookup/lung-cancer/saved-by-the-scan.
- "Lung Cancer Screening," U.S. Preventive Services Task Force (USPSTF), March 9, 2021, https://www.uspreventiveservicestaskforce.org/uspstf/recommendation/lung-cancer-screening.
- "What to Expect During a Skin Cancer Screening," American Society of Clinical Oncology (ASCO), May 31, 2022, https://www.cancer.net/blog/2022-05/what-expect-during-skin-cancer-screening.
- "Oral Cancer Screening," Mayo Clinic, October 30, 2021, https://www.mayoclinic.org/tests-procedures/oral-cancer-screening/about/pac-20394802.
- Christian Pavlovich, MD, "Prostate Cancer: Age-Specific Screening Guidelines," Johns Hopkins Medicine, accessed November 19, 2022, https://www.hopkinsmedicine.org/health/conditions-and-diseases/prostate-cancer/prostate-cancer-age-specific-screening-guidelines.

Videos
- Rangan Chatterjee, MD, "How to Make Diseases Disappear," TED Talk, June 2016, https://www.youtube.com/watch?v=gaY4m00wXpw.

CHAPTER 3

Choosing the Type of Doctor You Need
Articles
- Jennifer Berry, reviewed by Alana Biggers, "Types of Doctors and What They Do," Medical News Today, December 16, 2019, https://www.medicalnewstoday.com/articles/types-of-doctors.
- "Different Kinds of Doctors from A to Z," MDhealth.com, updated November 10, 2022, https://www.md-health.com/Types-Of-Doctors.html.
- Brunilda Nazario, "How to Choose a Doctor," WebMD, reviewed December 13, 2021, https://www.webmd.com/health-insurance/how-to-choose-a-doctor.
- Leah Alexander, "What Kind of Doctor Do I Need?" HealthPages.org, updated August 13, 2022, https://www.healthpages.org/health-care/what-kind-of-doctor-do-ineed/.
- "Choosing a Doctor: Quick Tips," Office of Disease Prevention and Health Promotion (OASH), U.S. Department of Health & Human Services, updated June 1, 2022, https://health.gov/myhealthfinder/doctor-visits/regular-checkups/choosing-doctor-quick-tips.

CHAPTER 4

Partnering with Your Doctor
Articles
- "Questions to Ask Your Doctor," MedicineNet, accessed November 19, 2022, https://www.medicinenet.com/questions_to_ask_your_doctor_-_general/views.htm.
- "Questions to Ask Your Health Care Team," CancerCare, updated June 24, 2022, https://www.cancercare.org/publications/243-questions_to_ask_your_health_care_team.
- "10 Questions to Ask Before Having an Operation," American College of Surgeons (ACS), accessed November 19, 2022, https://www.facs.org/for-patients/preparing-for-your-surgery/10-questions/.
- Jennifer Whitlock, reviewed by Jennifer Schwartz, fact checked by Nick Blackmer, "Important Questions to Ask Before You Have Surgery," Verywell Health, updated April 7, 2022, https://www.verywellhealth.com/surgery-questions-you-should-ask-3157021.

- Melinda Wenner Moyer, "Facing Surgery? Here's How to Prepare," *New York Times*, October 31, 2022, https://www.nytimes.com/2022/10/20/well/live/prepare-for-surgery.html.
- Z. Colette Edwards, "The Day After.... Cancer Survivorship," Wharton Health Care Management Alumni Association, *Wharton Healthcare Quarterly*, Winter 2020, https://www.whartonhealthcare.org/the_day_after_cancer_survivorship.
- "What Should I Ask My Doctor During a Checkup?," National Institute on Aging (NIA), National Institutes of Health (NIH), reviewed February 3, 2020, https://www.nia.nih.gov/health/what-should-i-ask-my-doctor-during-checkup.

CHAPTER 5

Coordinating Care

Articles
- The United Hospital Fund, "A Family Caregiver's Guide to Care Coordination," Next Step in Care, 2014, https://www.nextstepincare.org/uploads/File/Guides/Care_Coordination/Care_Coordination.pdf.
- "Care Coordination," Agency for Healthcare Research and Quality (AHRQ), reviewed August 2018, https://www.ahrq.gov/ncepcr/care/coordination.html.
- Bailey Gensley, "Tips & Tricks From Our Team: Staying on Top of Your Medications," Duos, September 19, 2022, https://www.getduos.com/blog-post/staying-on-top-of-your-medications.

Videos
- Atul Gawande, "How do we heal medicine?" TED Talk, March 2012, https://www.youtube.com/watch?v=L3QkaS249Bc.

CHAPTER 6

Having a Baby

Articles
- Jennifer Larson, reviewed by Laura K. Grubb, "8 questions to ask if you're planning a pregnancy," The Checkup by Single Care, July 19, 2021, https://www.singlecare.com/blog/questions-to-ask-doctor-before-getting-pregnant/.
- Updated by John D. Jacobson, reviewed by David Zieve, "Questions to ask your doctor about labor and delivery," MedlinePlus, National Library of Medicine (U.S.), reviewed June 30, 2020, https://medlineplus.gov/ency/patientinstructions/000960.htm.

- "Postpartum Depression," Mayo Clinic, May 24, 2022, https://www.mayoclinic.org/diseases-conditions/postpartum-depression/symptoms-causes/syc-20376617.

Websites
- "Clinical Guidance/Obstetric Care Consensus," American College of Obstetricians and Gynecologists (ACOG), accessed November 19, 2022, https://www.acog.org/clinical/clinical-guidance/obstetric-care-consensus.
- "On Your Parenting Journey Now? Find the Resources You Need," March of Dimes, accessed November 19, 2022, https://www.marchofdimes.org/.
- "Birth Equity for All Black Birthing People," National Birth Equity Collaborative (NBEC), 2022, https://birthequity.org/.
- Reviewed by John W. Schmitt, MD, "Prenatal Care," OASH/Office on Women's Health, U.S. Department of Health & Human Services, updated February 22, 2021, https://www.womenshealth.gov/a-z-topics/prenatal-care.

CHAPTER 7

Deciding Where to Go When a Medical Need Arises

Articles
- Nicole Pajer, "How to Find the Best Health Care in a Post-Pandemic World," AARP, May 9, 2022, https://www.aarp.org/health/conditions-treatments/info-2022/best-medical-care.html.

Websites
- "Find and Compare Nursing Homes, Hospitals, and Other Providers Near You," Medicare.gov, U.S. Centers for Medicare and Medicaid Services, accessed November 19, 2022, https://www.medicare.gov/care-compare/.
- "Find Doctors and Medical Facilities," USA.gov, https://www.usa.gov/doctors.
- "Feel Better About Finding Healthcare," Healthgrades, 2022, https://www.healthgrades.com/.
- "Information You Can Trust: Verify a Doctor's License and Professional Background Information," DocInfo, Federation of State Medical Boards (FSMB), accessed November 19, 2022, https://www.docinfo.org.

- "Find a Gold Seal Health Care Organization," Quality Check, The Joint Commission, accessed November 19, 2022, https://www.qualitycheck.org/.

CHAPTER 8

Maintaining Your Emotional Health

Articles
- "Racism and Mental Health," Mind, accessed November 19, 2022, https://www.mind.org.uk/information-support/tips-for-everyday-living/racism-and-mental-health/.
- Kendra Cherry, "Mental Health Resources to Support the LGBTQ+ Community," updated June 9, 2021, Verywell Mind, https://www.verywellmind.com/16-mental-health-resources-to-support-the-lgbtq-community-5188200.

Websites
- "The Go-To Solution for Mental Health Education and Connection," PsychHub, https://psychhub.com/.
- "55 Mental Health Resources for People of Color," Online MSW Programs, 2U Inc, https://www.onlinemswprograms.com/resources/mental-health-resources-racial-ethnic-groups/.
- "Mental Health," U.S. Department of Veterans Affairs, https://www.mentalhealth.va.gov/.
- "Help for Service Members and Their Families," MentalHealth.gov, updated March 1, 2022, https://www.mentalhealth.gov/get-help/veterans.

CHAPTER 9

Dealing with Mental Illness

- Suicide and Crisis Lifeline: Call or text 988, nationwide.

Articles
- Reviewed by Anthony T. Ng, "Warning Signs of Mental Illness," American Psychiatric Association, accessed November 19, 2022, https://www.psychiatry.org/patients-families/warning-signs-of-mental-illness.

Websites
- National Alliance on Mental Illness (NAMI), https://www.nami.org/Home.

- "The Go-To Solution for Mental Health Education and Connection," Psych Hub, https://psychhub.com/.
- Substance Abuse and Mental Health Services Administration (SAMHSA), https://www.samhsa.gov/.
- "Patients and Families," American Psychiatric Association (APA), https://www.psychiatry.org/patients-families.
- "Psychology Topics," American Psychological Association (APA), https://www.apa.org/topics.

CHAPTER 10

Facing Health Disparities

Books

- Marilyn Hughes Gaston, MD, and Gayle K. Porter, Psy.D., *Prime Time: The African American Woman's Complete Guide to Midlife Health and Wellness*, Orlando, Florida: Dare Books, 2001.
- Anushay Hossain, *The Pain Gap: How Sexism and Racism in Healthcare Kill Women*, New York: S&S/Simon Element, 2021.
- Victoria Holloway, Miss Diagnosed: *The Health Handbook Every Woman (and Man) Should Read*, United Kingdom: Livi, July 18, 2022, https://partners.livi.co.uk/hubfs/Livi_Miss_Diagnosed_eBook_digital.pdf.

Articles

- Erin Paterson, "Advocating for a Sick Parent by Confronting Physician Bias," KevinMD.com, MedPage Today, March 19, 2022, https://www.kevinmd.com/2022/03/advocating-for-a-sick-parent-by-confronting-physician-bias.html.
- Anna Smith, reviewed by Jason Daniel-Ulloa, "Biases in healthcare: An overview," *Medical News Today*, August 30, 2021, https://www.medicalnewstoday.com/articles/biases-in-healthcare.
- "Cancer Disparities," National Cancer Institute (NIH), reviewed March 28, 2022, https://www.cancer.gov/about-cancer/understanding/disparities.
- Nambi Ndugga and Samantha Artiga, "Disparities in Health and Health Care: 5 Key Questions and Answers," KFF, May 11, 2021, https://www.kff.org/racial-equity-and-health-policy/issue-brief/disparities-in-health-and-health-care-5-key-questions-and-answers/.
- "How To Protect Against Race and Gender Healthcare Bias," RocketLawyer, updated August 8, 2022, https://www.rocketlawyer.com/family-and-personal/health-and-medical/healthcare-decisions/legal-guide/how-to-protect-against-ace-and-gender-healthcare-bias.

- Aashna Gheewalla, reviewed by Alyssa Billingsley, "What Is Medical Gaslighting, and How Do You Know If It's Happening to You?," GoodRx Health, May 19, 2022, https://www.goodrx.com/healthcare-access/patient-advocacy/medical-gaslighting-signs-examples.
- Anahad O'Connor, "Why Heart Disease in Women Is So Often Missed or Dismissed," *New York Times*, May 9, 2022, https://nyti.ms/3kUwThy.
- "Cancer Disparities," National Cancer Institute (NCI), National Institutes of Health (NIH), reviewed March 28, 2022, https://www.cancer.gov/about-cancer/understanding/disparities.

Websites
- "Your First Stop for Rural Health Information," Rural Health Information Hub (RHIhub), https://ruralhealthinfo.org.
- World Professional Association for Transgender Health (WPATH), https://www.wpath.org/about/mission-and-vision.

Videos
- David R. Williams, "How Racism Makes Us Sick," TED Talk, November 2016, https://www.youtube.com/watch?v=VzyjDR_AWzE.

CHAPTER 11

Paying for Healthcare
- No Surprises Help Desk: 1-800-985-3059

Articles
- Melinda Wenner Moyer, "How to Dispute Surprise Medical Bills," *New York Times*, June 30, 2022, https://www.nytimes.com/2022/06/30/well/live/surprise-medical-bills.html.
- "A Healthcare Survival Guide for the Uninsured," Health Karma, February 2022, https://blog.healthkarma.org/a-healthcare-survival-guide-for-the-uninsured/?utm_sq=gz0vznfeih&page=1.
- Colin Bean, "What is Coordination of Benefits?" *eHealth*, updated September 15, 2022, https://www.ehealthinsurance.com/resources/individual-and-family/coordination-of-benefits.
- "Coordination of Benefits," CMS.gov, U.S. Centers for Medicare & Medicaid Services, modified December 1, 2021, https://www.cms.gov/Medicare/Coordination-of-Benefits-and-Recovery/Coordination-of-Benefits-and-Recovery-Overview/Coordination-of-Benefits/Coordination-of-Benefits.

- "Coordination of Benefits & Third Party Liability," Medicaid.gov, U.S. Centers for Medicare & Medicaid Services, accessed November 19, 2022, https://www.medicaid.gov/medicaid/eligibility/coordination-of-benefits-third-party-liability/index.html.
- "Medicare Resource Center," AARP, accessed November 19, 2022, https://www.aarp.org/health/medicare-insurance/.

Websites
- "Find Your Most Affordable Health Plan," Health Sherpa, https://www.healthsherpa.com/.
- HealthCare.gov, https://www.healthcare.gov/.
- CMS.gov, U.S. Centers for Medicare & Medicaid Services, https://CMS.gov.
- "On Your Side Through Life's Financial Moments," Consumer Financial Protection Bureau (CFPB): https://www.consumerfinance.gov/.

CHAPTER 12

Preparing for the End of Life

Books
- BJ Miller, MD, and Shoshana Berger, *A Beginner's Guide to the End: Practical Advice for Living Life and Facing Death*, New York: Simon & Schuster, 2019.
- Atul Gawande, *Being Mortal: Medicine and What Matters in the End*, New York: Henry Holt & Company, 2014.
- Paul Kalanithi, *When Breath Becomes Air*, New York: Random House, 2016.

Articles
- Rachael Bedard, "What My Grandmother Knew About Dying," *The New Yorker*, March 6, 2022, https://www-newyorker-com.cdn.ampproject.org/c/s/www.newyorker.com/culture/personal-history/what-my-grandmother-knew-about-dying/amp.
- "5 commonly held myths about end-of-life issues," Harvard Health Publishing, Harvard Medical School, August 25, 2022, https://www.health.harvard.edu/diseases-and-conditions/5-commonly-held-myths-about-end-of-life-issues.
- "End-of-life planning checklist: A guide to the 12 documents you should consider," *Freewill*, updated March 1, 2022, https://www.freewill.com/learn/end-of-life-planning-checklist.

- Kathleen Davis, reviewed by Shilpa Amin, "What to know about end-of-life planning," Medical News Today, October 11, 2021, https://www.medicalnewstoday.com/articles/end-of-life-planning#what-to-expect.
- Amy Goyer and Andy Markowitz, "How to Start a Conversation About End-of-Life Care," AARP Family Caregiving, updated October 14, 2021, https://www.aarp.org/caregiving/basics/info-2020/end-of-life-talk-care-talk.html.

Websites
- "Five Wishes," https://www.fivewishes.org/.
- "Resources for End-of-Life Planning and Care," International Children's Palliative Care Network (ICPCN), https://www.icpcn.org/resources-for-end-of-life-planning-and-care/.

Guide to Acronyms & Abbreviations

AA	Alcoholics Anonymous
AAFP	American Academy of Family Physicians
AAIP	Association of American Indian Physicians
AAPA	American Academy of Physician Associates
AATA	American Art Therapy Association
ABV	alcohol by volume
ACA	Affordable Care Act
ACOG	American College of Obstetricians and Gynecologists
ADA	Americans with Disabilities Act
ADFMs	active-duty family members
ADHD	attention deficit hyperactivity disorder
ADLs	activities of daily living
ADSMs	active-duty service members
ADTA	American Dance Therapy Association
Afib	atrial fibrillation
ALS	amyotrophic lateral sclerosis (aka Lou Gehrig's Disease)
ARC	Appalachian Regional Commission
BHP	Basic Health Program
BMI	body mass index
BPD	borderline personality disorder
CA 19-9	cancer antigen 19-9 blood test
CAPC	Center to Advance Palliative Care
CBT	cognitive behavioral therapy
CCRC	Continuing Care Retirement Community
CCU	cardiac care unit
CDC	Centers for Disease Control and Prevention
C. diff	*Clostridium difficile*

CEO	Chief Executive Officer
CHIP	Children's Health Insurance Program
COB	coordination of benefits
COBRA	Consolidated Omnibus Budget Reconciliation Act
COE	Center of Excellence
COPD	chronic obstructive pulmonary disease
CRP	C-reactive protein
CSB	Community Services Board
C-section	Cesarean section
CT scan	computerized tomography scan
D&C	dilation and curettage
DDS	Doctor of Dental Surgery
DHMO	Dental Health Maintenance Organization
DMD	Doctor of Medicine in Dentistry
DME	durable medical equipment
DMHAS	Division of Mental Health and Addiction Services
DMO	Dental Maintenance Organization
DNA	deoxyribonucleic acid
DNR	Do Not Resuscitate
DO	Doctor of Osteopathic Medicine
DOL	Department of Labor
DONA	Doulas of North America (formerly)
EAP	employee assistance program
EEG	electroencephalogram
EFT	emotional freedom technique
EHR	electronic health record
EKG	electrocardiogram
EMDR	eye movement desensitization and reprocessing
EMR	electronic medical record
EMT	emergency medical technician
EMTALA	Emergency Medical Treatment & Labor Act
ENT	ear, nose, and throat specialist
EOB	Explanation of Benefits
ER	emergency room
ESR	erythrocyte sedimentation rate
ESRD	end-stage renal disease

FDA	Food and Drug Administration
FDIC	Federal Deposit Insurance Corporation
FMLA	Family Medical Leave Act
FQHC	Federally Qualified Health Center
FSA	Flexible Spending Account
GDP	gross domestic product
GERD	gastroesophageal reflux disease
GI	gastrointestinal
GLMA	Health Professionals Advancing LGBTQ Equality (formerly Gay & Lesbian Medical Association)
GMO	genetically modified organism
HDHP	high deductible health plan
HG	hyperemesis gravidarum
HHS	Health and Human Services
HIPAA	Health Insurance Portability and Accountability Act
HIV/AIDS	human immunodeficiency virus/acquired immunodeficiency syndrome
HMO	health maintenance organization
HOPD	hospital outpatient department
HPV	human papillomavirus
HR	human resources
HRA	Health Reimbursement Account
HRSA	Health Resources and Services Administration
HRT	hormone replacement therapy
HSA	Health Savings Account
ICU	intensive care unit
IFEC	independent freestanding emergency center
IUI	intrauterine insemination
IV	intravenous
IVF	in vitro fertilization
JAMA	*Journal of the American Medical Association*
LGBTQIA+	lesbian, gay, bisexual, transgender, queer, intersex, asexual, and others
LTC	long-term care
LTD	long-term disability

MA	Medicare Advantage
MBSR	Mindfulness-Based Stress Reduction
MD	Doctor of Medicine
MHS	Military Health System
MRI	magnetic resonance imaging
MRSA	methicillin-resistant *Staphylococcus aureus* infection
MS	multiple sclerosis
MSP	Medicare Savings Programs
MUA	Medically Underserved Area
MUP	Medically Underserved Population
NACPM	National Association of Certified Professional Midwives
NAMI	National Alliance on Mental Illness
NCAPIP	National Council of Asian Pacific Islander Physicians
NCCIH	National Center for Complementary and Integrative Health
NHMA	National Hispanic Medical Association
NHPCO	National Hospice and Palliative Care Organization
NICU	neonatal intensive care unit
NIH	National Institutes of Health
NIHCM	National Institute for Health Care Management
NIMH	National Institute of Mental Health
NIPS	noninvasive prenatal screening
NIPT	noninvasive prenatal tests
NMA	National Medical Association
NP	nurse practitioner
NPCRC	National Palliative Care Research Center
OB/GYN	obstetrician/gynecologist
OCD	obsessive compulsive disorder
OECD	Organization for Economic Cooperation and Development
OIG	Office of Inspector General
OTC	over-the-counter
PA	physician assistant/associate
PACT	Program of Assertive Community Treatment
Pap smear	Papanicolaou test

PCOS	polycystic ovary syndrome
PCP	primary care physician (practitioner)
PFAC	Patient and Family Advisory Council
PICC line	peripherally inserted central catheter line
PKU	phenylketonuria
PPO	preferred provider organization
PSA	prostate-specific antigen
PT	physical therapy
PTSD	post-traumatic stress disorder
PUA	Pandemic Unemployment Assistance
R&C	reasonable and customary
RN	registered nurse
SAMHSA	Substance Abuse and Mental Health Services Administration
SHOP	Small Business Health Options Program
SIDS	sudden infant death syndrome
SNP	Special Needs Plan
SPD	summary plan description
SSDI	Social Security Disability Insurance
SSI	Supplemental Security Income
STD	short-term disability
TAVR	transcatheter aortic valve replacement
TBI	traumatic brain injury
TPN	total parenteral nutrition
U&C	usual and customary
U&P	usual and prevailing
USPHS	United States Public Health Service
UTI	urinary tract infection
VBAC	vaginal birth after cesarean
V-tach	ventricular tachycardia

Endnotes

CHAPTER 2

Embracing a Healthier Lifestyle

1 "American Cancer Society Prevention and Early Detection Guidelines," American Cancer Society, accessed November 19, 2022, https://www.cancer.org/health-care-professionals/american-cancer-society-prevention-early-detection-guidelines.html.

2 "Breast Cancer in Men," Centers for Disease Control and Prevention, Division of Cancer Prevention and Control, last reviewed September 26, 2022, https://www.cdc.gov/cancer/breast/men/index.htm.

3 Leiyu Shi, "The Impact of Primary Care: A Focused Review," National Library of Medicine, published online December 31, 2012, https://www.ncbi.nlm.nih.gov/pmc/articles/PMC3820521/.

4 Andis Robeznieks, "Doctor Shortages Are Here—and They'll Get Worse If We Don't Act Fast," AMA, April 13, 2022, https://www.ama-assn.org/practice-management/sustainability/doctor-shortages-are-here-and-they-ll-get-worse-if-we-don-t-act.

5 Meg Bryant, "Nurse Practitioners Increasingly Fill Gap in Primary Care Delivery, Study Finds," *HealthCare Dive*, June 5, 2018, https://www.healthcaredive.com/news/nurse-practitioners-increasingly-fill-gap-in-primary-care-delivery-study-f/524961/.

6 "The Surprising Connections Between Oral Health and Well Being," University of Illinois at Chicago College of Dentistry, January 14, 2019, https://dentistry.uic.edu/news-stories/the-surprising-connections-between-oral-health-and-well-being/.

7 "Health and Economic Costs of Chronic Diseases," National Center for Chronic Disease Prevention and Health Promotion (NCCDPHP), Centers for Disease Control and Prevention (CDC), last reviewed September 8, 2022, https://www.cdc.gov/chronicdisease/about/costs/index.htm.

8 "Per capita health expenditures in selected countries in 2020 (in U.S. dollars)," *Statista*, November 11, 2022, https://www.statista.com/statistics/236541/per-capita-health-expenditure-by-country/.

9 "Results from the Annual National Youth Tobacco Survey," U.S. Food & Drug Administration (FDA), November 10, 2022, https://www.fda.gov/tobacco-products/youth-and-tobacco/results-annual-national-youth-tobacco-survey.

10 "Health Benefits of Quitting Smoking Over Time," American Cancer Society, last reviewed November 10, 2020, https://www.cancer.org/healthy/stay-away-from-tobacco/benefits-of-quitting-smoking-over-time.html.

11 "About Chronic Diseases," National Center for Chronic Disease Prevention and Health Promotion (NCCDPHP), Centers for Disease Control and Prevention (CDC), last reviewed July 21, 2022, https://www.cdc.gov/chronicdisease/about/index.htm.

12 "Adult Obesity Facts," Division of Nutrition, Physical Activity, and Obesity, Centers for Disease Control and Prevention (CDC), last reviewed May 17, 2022, https://www.cdc.gov/obesity/data/adult.html.

13 Ruairi Robertson, "Why the Gut Microbiome is Crucial for Your Health," *Healthline*, updated June 27, 2017, https://www.healthline.com/nutrition/gut-microbiome-and-health.

14 Kris Gunnars and Rachael Link, reviewed by Kim Chin, "Mediterranean Diet 101: A Meal Plan and Beginner's Guide," *Healthline*, updated October 25, 2021, https://www.healthline.com/nutrition/mediterranean-diet-meal-plan.

15 "For cancer prevention, it's best not to drink alcohol," American Institute for Cancer Research, accessed November 19, 2022, https://www.aicr.org/cancer-prevention/recommendations/limit-alcohol-consumption/.

16 "Alcohol Use and Your Health," Centers for Disease Control and Prevention (CDC), last reviewed April 14, 2022, https://www.cdc.gov/alcohol/fact-sheets/alcohol-use.htm.

17 Shaojuan Hu, Lorelei Tucker, Chongyun Wu, Luodan Yang, "Beneficial Effects of Exercise on Depression and Anxiety During the Covid-19 Pandemic: A Narrative Review," *Frontiers in Psychiatry*, November 4, 2020, https://www.frontiersin.org/articles/10.3389/fpsyt.2020.587557/full.

18 London School of Hygiene & Tropical Medicine (LSHTM), "Light and moderate physical activity reduces the risk of early death, study finds," *ScienceDaily*, July 25, 2010, accessed November 12, 2022, https://www.sciencedaily.com/releases/2010/07/100723112713.htm.

ENDNOTES

19 "1 in 3 adults don't get enough sleep," Centers for Disease Control and Prevention (CDC), last reviewed February 16, 2016, https://www.cdc.gov/media/releases/2016/p0215-enough-sleep.html.

20 Eric Suni, reviewed by Abhinav Singh, "Sleep Apnea," Sleep Foundation, updated October 19, 2022, https://www.sleepfoundation.org/sleep-apnea.

21 Alison Caldwell, "Getting more sleep reduces caloric intake, a game change for weight loss programs," University of Chicago Medicine, February 7, 2022, https://www.uchicagomedicine.org/forefront/research-and-discoveries-articles/getting-more-sleep-reduces-caloric-intake.

22 Zawn Villines, reviewed by Heidi Moawad, "Serotonin deficiency: Symptoms and treatment," *Medical News Today*, October 5, 2022, https://www.medicalnewstoday.com/articles/serotonin-deficiency.

23 "Shift Work Sleep Disorder," Cleveland Clinic, last reviewed February 25, 2021, https://my.clevelandclinic.org/health/diseases/12146-shift-work-sleep-disorder.

CHAPTER 3

Choosing the Type of Doctor You Need

1 Brent A. Bauer, MD, "What kind of doctor is a D.O.? Does a D.O. have the same training as an M.D.?," Consumer Health, Mayo Clinic, February 9, 2021, https://www.mayoclinic.org/healthy-lifestyle/consumer-health/expert-answers/osteopathic-medicine/faq-20058168.

2 "Complementary, Alternative, or Integrative Health: What's In A Name?," National Center for Complementary and Integrative Health, last updated April 2021, https://www.nccih.nih.gov/health/complementary-alternative-or-integrative-health-whats-in-a-name.

3 Mayo Clinic Staff, "Oral Health: A window to your overall health," *Adult Health*, Mayo Clinic, October 28, 2021, https://www.mayoclinic.org/healthy-lifestyle/adult-health/in-depth/dental/art-20047475.

CHAPTER 4

Partnering with Your Doctor

1 Jennifer Fong Ha and Nancy Longnecker, "Doctor-Patient Communication: A Review," *Ochsner Journal*, Spring 2010, National Library of Medicine, https://www.ncbi.nlm.nih.gov/pmc/articles/PMC3096184/.

2 "Adverse Events in Hospitals: A Quarter of Medicare Patients Experienced Harm in October 2018," Office of Inspector General, U.S. Department of Health and Human Services, May 9, 2022, https://oig.hhs.gov/oei/reports/OEI-06-18-00400.asp.
3 "Adverse Events," Office of Inspector General, U.S. Department of Health and Human Services, June 16, 2022, https://oig.hhs.gov/reports-and-publications/featured-topics/adverse-events.

CHAPTER 5

Coordinating Care

1 "Medication overload and older Americans," Lown Institute, accessed November 19, 2022, https://lowninstitute.org/projects/medication-overload-how-the-drive-to-prescribe-is-harming-older-americans/.
2 "What is Care Coordination?," *NEJM Catalyst Innovations in Care Delivery*, January 1, 2018, https://catalyst.nejm.org/doi/full/10.1056/CAT.18.0291.

CHAPTER 6

Having a Baby

1 Bekir Kahveci, Rauf Melekoglu, Ismail Cuneyt Evruke, and Cehan Cetin, "The effect of advanced maternal age on perinatal outcomes in nulliparous singleton pregnancies," *BMC Pregnancy and Childbirth*, August 22, 2018, https://bmcpregnancychildbirth.biomedcentral.com/articles/10.1186/s12884-018-1984-x.
2 Roosa Tikkanen, Munira Z. Gunja, Molly FitzGerald, and Laurie Zephyrin, "Maternal Mortality and Maternity Care in the United States Compared to 10 Other Developed Countries," The Commonwealth Fund, November 18, 2020, https://www.commonwealthfund.org/publications/issue-briefs/2020/nov/maternal-mortality-maternity-care-us-compared-10-countries.
3 Donna L. Hoyert, "Maternal Mortality Rates in the United States, 2020," National Center for Health Statistics, Centers for Disease Control and Prevention (CDC), last reviewed February 23, 2022, https://www.cdc.gov/nchs/data/hestat/maternal-mortality/2020/maternal-mortality-rates-2020.htm.
4 "Male Infertility," Cleveland Clinic, last reviewed May 26, 2021, https://my.clevelandclinic.org/health/diseases/17201-male-infertility.

5 Reviewed by Esther Eisenberg, Kelly Brumbaugh, Renee Brown-Bryant, and Lee Warner, "Infertility," Office on Women's Health, last updated February 22, 2021, https://www.womenshealth.gov/a-z-topics/infertility.

6 "How common is male infertility, and what are its causes?," National Institute of Child Health and Human Development (NICHD), last reviewed November 18, 2021, https://www.nichd.nih.gov/health/topics/menshealth/conditioninfo/infertility.

7 Stephanie Watson, reviewed by Hansa D. Bhargava, "Same-Sex Couples Face Fertility Issues When Trying to Conceive," *WebMD*, December 16, 2020, https://www.webmd.com/infertility-and-reproduction/features/same-sex-couples-pregnancy.

8 Jessica N. Sanders, Sara E. Simonsen, Christina A. Porucznik, Ahmad O. Hammoud, Ken Smith, and Joseph Stanford, "Fertility Treatments and the Risk of Preterm Birth Among Women with Subfertility: A Linked-Data Retrospective Cohort Study," Research Square, February 12, 2021, https://assets.researchsquare.com/files/rs-206714/v1/fa2443c6-8c4a-4930-b94d-121418d3f6f5.pdf?c=1648562288.

9 "FDA Warns of Risks Associated with Non-Invasive Prenatal Screening Tests," U.S. Food and Drug Administration (FDA), April 19, 2022, https://www.fda.gov/news-events/press-announcements/fda-warns-risks-associated-non-invasive-prenatal-screening-tests.

10 Mayo Clinic Staff, "Miscarriage," Mayo Clinic, accessed November 19, 2022, https://www.mayoclinic.org/diseases-conditions/pregnancy-loss-miscarriage/symptoms-causes/syc-20354298.

11 Huifeng Shi, Lian Chen, Yuanyuan Wang, et al., "Severity of Anemia During Pregnancy and Adverse Maternal and Fetal Outcomes," JAMA Network, February 3, 2022, https://jamanetwork.com/journals/jamanetworkopen/fullarticle/2788631.

12 "Gestational Diabetes," March of Dimes, last reviewed March 2022, https://www.marchofdimes.org/complications/gestational-diabetes.aspx.

13 "Preeclampsia," March of Dimes, reviewed October 2020, https://www.marchofdimes.org/complications/preeclampsia.aspx.

14 "Births—Method of Delivery," National Center for Health Statistics, Centers for Disease Control and Prevention (CDC), last reviewed May 16, 2022, https://www.cdc.gov/nchs/fastats/delivery.htm.

15 Joyce A. Martin, Brady E. Hamilton, and Michelle J.K. Osterman, "Births in the United States, 2020," National Center for Health Statistics, Centers for Disease Control and Prevention (CDC), September 2021, https://www.cdc.gov/nchs/products/databriefs/db418.htm.

16 "Low-risk Cesarean Delivery," *America's Health Rankings*, accessed November 19, 2022, https://www.americashealthrankings.org/explore/health-of-women-and-children/measure/low_risk_cesarean/state/ALL.

17 "Vaginal Birth After Cesarean: VBAC," American Pregnancy Association, accessed November 19, 2022, https://americanpregnancy.org/healthy-pregnancy/labor-and-birth/vaginal-birth-after-cesarean/.

18 Debra Fulghum Bruce, reviewed by Traci C. Johnson, "Postpartum Depression," WebMD, reviewed August 23, 2022, https://www.webmd.com/depression/guide/postpartum-depression.

19 "Cost of Having a Baby – Full Overview of Childbirth Expenses," Balancing Everything, December 31, 2021, https://balancingeverything.com/cost-of-having-a-baby/.

20 Andrew Hurst, "The Cost of a C-Section Is More Than $9,000 Greater on Average Than a Vaginal Delivery," Value Penguin, updated May 3, 2021, https://www.valuepenguin.com/cost-of-vaginal-births-vs-c-sections.

21 "Cost of Having a Baby – Full Overview of Childbirth Expenses," Balancing Everything, December 31, 2021, https://balancingeverything.com/cost-of-having-a-baby/.

22 David Weliver, "The Real Cost of Having a Baby," Money Under 30, modified June 2, 2022, https://www.moneyunder30.com/cost-of-having-a-baby.

CHAPTER 7

Deciding Where to Go When a Medical Need Arises

1 Rachael Lau and Rachael Lau, "Federally Qualified Health Center (FQHC)," American Pharmacists, accessed January 11, 2023, Association, https://www.pharmacist.com/Practice/Practice-Resources/Learn-the-Lingo/federally-qualified-health-center-fqhc

2 Sam Whitehead, "Turned Away from Urgent Care—And Toward a Big ED Bill," Medscape, October 3, 2022, https://www.medscape.com/viewarticle/981800.

3 Elizabeth Davis, RN, "What is Hospital Observation Status? Not All Hospital Stays Are Considered Inpatient Care," Verywell Health, updated on April 27, 2022, https://www.verywellhealth.com/what-is-hospital-observation-status-1738754.

4   "2021 Walmart Centers of Excellence," accessed November 19, 2022, https://one.walmart.com/content/dam/themepage/pdfs/centers-of-excellence-overview-2021.pdf.

CHAPTER 8

Maintaining Your Emotional Health

1   Catherine K. Ettman, Salma M. Abdalla, Gregory H. Cohen, et al., "Prevalence of Depression Symptoms in U.S. Adults Before and During the COVID-19 Pandemic," JAMA Network, September 2, 2020, https://jamanetwork.com/journals/jamanetworkopen/fullarticle/2770146.

2   Nick Tate, reviewed by Brunilda Nazario, "Loneliness Rivals Obesity, Smoking, as Health Risk," WebMD, reviewed May 4, 2018, https://www.webmd.com/balance/news/20180504/loneliness-rivals-obesity-smoking-as-health-risk.

3   Joshua Schultz, reviewed by Jo Nash, "5 Differences Between Mindfulness and Meditation," PositivePsychology.com, July 24, 2020, https://positivepsychology.com/differences-between-mindfulness-meditation/.

4   The American Dance Therapy Association (ADTA), "Frequently Asked Questions," accessed on January 11, 2023, https://www.adta.org/become-a-dance-movement-therapist.

CHAPTER 9

Dealing with Mental Illness

1   "Mental Health By the Numbers," National Alliance on Mental Illness (NAMI), last updated June 2022, https://nami.org/mhstats.

2   "The Ripple Effect of Mental Illness," National Alliance on Mental Illness (NAMI), accessed November 19, 2022, https://stage.nami.org/NAMI/media/NAMI-Media/Infographics/NAMI_Impact_RippleEffect_2020_FINAL.pdf.

3   "Eating Disorders in Men & Boys," National Eating Disorders Association (NEDA), accessed November 19, 2022, https://www.nationaleatingdisorders.org/learn/general-information/research-on-males.

4   "Schizophrenia Symptoms, Patterns and Statistics and Patterns," MentalHelp.net, accessed November 19, 2022, https://www.mentalhelp.net/schizophrenia/statistics/.

5 "Drug Overdose Deaths in the U.S. Top 100,000 Annually," National Center for Health Statistics, Centers for Disease Control and Prevention (CDC), last reviewed November 17, 2021, https://www.cdc.gov/nchs/pressroom/nchs_press_releases/2021/20211117.htm.

6 "Solutions & Challenges for Children's Mental Health in the COVID-19 Pandemic," National Institute for Health Care Management (NIHCM), 2021 update, https://infogram.com/1pkgxx2d6nrwedt9v9e623q5n5h3eq3p5qw.

CHAPTER 10

Facing Health Disparities

1 Kiara Taylor, reviewed by Erika Rasure, "The Digital Divide: What It Is, and What's Being Done To Close It," Investopedia, April 15, 2022, https://www.investopedia.com/the-digital-divide-5116352.

2 Jeremy Ney, "Food Deserts and Inequality," Social Policy Data Lab, September 30, 2021, https://www.socialpolicylab.org/post/grow-your-blog-community.

3 "State of Obesity 2022: Better Policies for a Healthier America," Trust for America's Health, September 27, 2022, https://www.tfah.org/report-details/state-of-obesity-2022/.

4 "Number of States with High Rates of Adult Obesity More Than Doubles," CDC Newsroom, last reviewed September 27, 2022, https://www.cdc.gov/media/releases/2022/p0927-states-obesity.html.

5 "The Tuskegee Timeline," The U.S. Public Health Service Syphilis Study at Tuskegee, CDC, last reviewed April 22, 2021, https://www.cdc.gov/tuskegee/timeline.htm.

6 Latoya Hill and Samantha Artiga, "Race/Ethnicity: Current Data and Changes Over Time," KFF, August 22, 2022, https://www.kff.org/coronavirus-covid-19/issue-brief/covid-19-cases-and-deaths-by-race-ethnicity-current-data-and-changes-over-time/.

7 Ryan K. Masters, Laudan Y. Aron, and Steven H. Woolf, "Changes in Life Expectancy Between 2019 and 2021: United States and 19 Peer Countries," medRxiv, April 7, 2022, https://www.medrxiv.org/content/10.1101/2022.04.05.22273393v1.

8 "Infant Mortality and African Americans," Office of Minority Health (OMH), U.S. Department of Health and Human Services, last modified July 8, 2021, https://www.minorityhealth.hhs.gov/omh/browse.aspx?lvl=4&lvlid=23.

9 "Minority Population Profiles," Office of Minority Health (OMH), U.S. Department of Health and Human Services, last modified October 12, 2021, https://minorityhealth.hhs.gov/omh/browse.aspx?lvl=2&lvlid=26.

10 Melanie Carver, Hannah Jaffee, Sanaz Eftekhari, and Mo Mayrides, "2020 Asthma Disparities in America," Asthma and Allergy Foundation of America (AAFA), accessed January 11, 2023, https://issuu.com/aafa.org/docs/asthma-disparities-in-america-burden-on-racial-eth

11 Brad N. Greenwood, Rachel R. Hardeman, Laura Huang, and Aaron Sojourner, "Physician–patient racial concordance and disparities in birthing mortality for newborns," *Proceedings of the National Academy of Sciences of the United State of America* (PNAS), August 17, 2020, https://www.pnas.org/doi/10.1073/pnas.1913405117.

12 "Lesbians and Cancer," National LGBT Cancer Network, https://cancer-network.org/cancer-information/lesbians-and-cancer/.

13 Anuradha Jetty, Yalda Jabbarpour, Jack Pollack, Ryan Huerto, Stephanie Woo, and Stephen Petterson, "Patient-Physician Racial Concordance Associated with Improved Healthcare Use and Lower Healthcare Expenditures in Minority Populations," *Springer Link*, February 24, 2021, https://link.springer.com/article/10.1007/s40615-020-00930-4.

14 Junko Takeshita, Shiyu Wang, and Alison W. Loren, et al., "Association of Racial/Ethnic and Gender Concordance Between Patients and Physicians With Patient Experience Ratings, JAMA Network, November 9, 2020, https://jamanetwork.com/journals/jamanetworkopen/fullarticle/2772682.

15 "Profile: Native Hawaiians/Pacific Islanders," Office of Minority Health (OMH), U.S. Department of Health and Human Services, last modified October 12, 2021, https://minorityhealth.hhs.gov/omh/browse.aspx?lvl=3&lvlid=65.

16 News@TheU, "Research identifies gender bias in estimation of patients' pain," University of Miami, April 6, 2021, https://news.miami.edu/stories/2021/04/research-identifies-gender-bias-in-estimation-of-patients-pain.html.

CHAPTER 11

Paying for Healthcare

1 "Health Coverage Changes Under the Affordable Care Act: End of 2021 Update," Issue Brief, Office of Health Policy, April 29, 2022, https://aspe.hhs.gov/sites/default/files/documents/77ba3e9c99264d4f76dd662d3b2498c0/aspe-ib-uninsured-aca.pdf.

2 "Economic Well-Being of U.S. Households (SHED): Dealing with Unexpected Expenses," Board of Governors of the Federal Reserve System, last updated August 22, 2022, https://www.federalreserve.gov/publications/2022-economic-well-being-of-us-households-in-2021-dealing-with-unexpected-expenses.htm.

3 Noam N. Levey, "100 Million People in America Are Saddled With Health Care Debt," KHN, June 16, 2022, https://khn.org/news/article/diagnosis-debt-investigation-100-million-americans-hidden-medical-debt/.

4 Hillary Hoffower, "Staggering medical bills are the biggest driver of personal bankruptcies in the U.S. Here's what you need to know if you're thinking about filing for bankruptcy," Insider, June 25, 2019, https://www.businessinsider.com/causes-personal-bankruptcy-medical-bills-mortgages-student-loan-debt-2019-6.

5 "How does health spending in the U.S. compare to other countries?," KFF, January 21, 2022, https://www.kff.org/slideshow/health-spending-in-the-u-s-as-compared-to-other-countries-slideshow/.

6 "Health Spending Indicator," OECD Data, accessed on November 13, 2022, https://data.oecd.org/healthres/health-spending.htm.

7 Brian McNeill, "U.S. life expectancy continued to fall in 2021," Virginia Commonwealth University, VCU News, April 7, 2022, https://www.news.vcu.edu/article/2022/04/us-life-expectancy-continued-to-fall-in-2021.

8 Roosa Tikkanen, Munira Z. Gunja, Molly FitzGerald, and Laurie Zephyrin, "Maternal Mortality and Maternity Care in the United States Compared to 10 Other Developed Countries," The Commonwealth Fund, November 18, 2020, https://www.commonwealthfund.org/publications/issue-briefs/2020/nov/maternal-mortality-maternity-care-us-compared-10-countries.

9 Roosa Tikkanen and Melinda K. Abrams, "U.S. Health Care from a Global Perspective, 2019: Higher Spending, Worse Outcomes?," The Commonwealth Fund Data Brief, January 2020, https://www.commonwealthfund.org/sites/default/files/2020-01/Tikkanen_US_hlt_care_global_perspective_2019_OECD_db_v2.pdf.

10 Matthew Rae, Gary Claxton, Krutika Amin, Emma Wager, Jared Ortaliza, and Cynthia Cox, "The Burden of Medical Debt in the United States," KFF, March 10, 2022, https://www.kff.org/health-costs/issue-brief/the-burden-of-medical-debt-in-the-united-states/.

11 Equifax, Inc., "Equifax, Experian, and TransUnion Support U.S. Consumers With Changes to Medical Collection Debt Reporting," CISION: PR Newswire, March 18, 2022, https://www.prnewswire.com/news-releases/equifax-experian-and-transunion-support-us-consumers-with-changes-to-medical-collection-debt-reporting-301505822.html.

ENDNOTES

12 "2021 Employer Health Benefits Survey—Section 1: Cost of Health Insurance," KFF, November 10, 2021, https://www.kff.org/health-costs/report/2021-employer-health-benefits-survey/.

13 Jamie Cattanach, "High-Deductible Health Plans Continue to Grow in Popularity, but Are They Right for You?" Value Penguin | Lending Tree, updated January 24, 2022, https://www.valuepenguin.com/high-deductible-health-plan-study

14 "High deductible health plan (HDHP)," HealthCare.gov, accessed November 19, 2022, https://www.healthcare.gov/glossary/high-deductible-health-plan/.

15 Centers for Medicare & Medicaid Services, "Health Reimbursement Arrangements," accessed January 13, 2023, https://www.cms.gov/cciio/programs-and-initiatives/health-insurance-market-reforms/health-reimbursement-arrangements

16 The Health Policy Institute, Georgetown University McCourt School of Public Policy, "Prescription Drugs, accessed January 13, 2023, https://hpi.georgetown.edu/rxdrugs/.

17 Meredith Freed, Jeannie Fuglesten Biniek, Anthony Damico, and Tricia Neuman, "Medicare Advantage in 2022: Enrollment Update and Key Trends," KFF, August 25, 2022, https://www.kff.org/medicare/issue-brief/medicare-advantage-in-2021-enrollment-update-and-key-trends/.

18 American Medical Association, "Understanding the Affordable Care Act," accessed January 13, 2023, https://www.ama-assn.org/delivering-care/patient-support-advocacy/understanding-affordable-care-act

19 Healthcare.gov, "The Children's Health Insurance Program (CHIP)," accessed January 13, 2023, https://www.healthcare.gov/medicaid-chip/childrens-health-insurance-program/

20 TRICARE, "Tricare 101," accessed January 13, 2023, https://www.tricare.mil/Plans/New?

21 Helen Leask, "Appeals Against Medical Insurance Denials Underused, Says Lawyer," Medscape, March 28, 2022, https://www.medscape.com/viewarticle/971008.

22 "Medical Debt Burden in the United States," Consumer Financial Protection Bureau (CFPB), February 2022, https://files.consumerfinance.gov/f/documents/cfpb_medical-debt-burden-in-the-united-states_report_2022-03.pdf.

23 Centers for Medicare & Medicaid, "Ending Surprise Medical Bills," accessed January 16, 2023, https://www.cms.gov/nosurprises

CHAPTER 12
Preparing for the End of Life

1. "2021 Senior Report," America's Health Rankings, accessed November 19, 2022, https://www.americashealthrankings.org/learn/reports/2021-senior-report/introduction.

2. William E. Gibson, "Age 65+ Adults are Projected to Outnumber Children by 2030," AARP Home and Family, March 14, 2018, https://www.aarp.org/home-family/friends-family/info-2018/census-baby-boomers-fd.html.

3. "National Health & Aging Trends Study (NHATS): How Daily Life Changes As We Age," National Study of Caregiving (NSOC), accessed November 19, 2022, https://www.nhats.org.

4. "Future Directions for the Demography of Aging: Proceedings of a Workshop," National Academies of Sciences, Engineering, and Medicine, 2018. https://nap.nationalacademies.org/catalog/25064/future-directions-for-the-demography-of-aging-proceedings-of-a.

5. "Life Expectancy in the U.S. Dropped for the Second Year in a Row in 2021," National Center for Health Statistics, Centers for Disease Control and Prevention (CDC), last reviewed August 31, 2022, https://www.cdc.gov/nchs/pressroom/nchs_press_releases/2022/20220831.htm.

6. "America's Care of Serious Illness: 2019 State-by-State Report Card on Access to Palliative Care in Our Nation's Hospitals," Center to Advance Palliative Care (CAPC), accessed November 19, 2022, https://reportcard.capc.org/.

7. "NHPCO Facts and Figures, 2021 Edition," National Hospice and Palliative Care Organization (NHPCO), October 2021, https://wpln.org/wp-content/uploads/sites/7/2021/12/NHPCO-Facts-Figures-2021-edition-1.pdf#page=9.

About the Authors

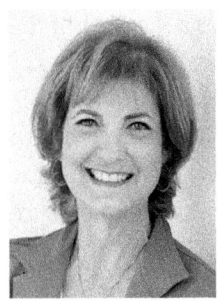

Charlene Rothkopf held a variety of corporate human resource positions with a global, multinational hospitality company, where she provided leadership to the health and welfare benefits department and led the implementation of the company's first corporate wellness program. Charlene then served as the senior human resource executive at a leading, publicly held, real estate development company.

Her lengthy journey as a patient navigating the healthcare system led her to pursue a coaching certificate from the Maryland University of Integrative Health and to establish the Wellness Consulting Group, LLC, an executive coaching and consulting firm specializing in executive and leadership development and organizational health and well-being. As a volunteer, Charlene has served as the co-lead of the Patient and Family Advisory Council for a major hospital system with the goal of bringing the patient's voice to hospital operations.

She currently resides in suburban Maryland, where she enjoys playing golf with her husband of over fifty years and spending time with her grandchildren.

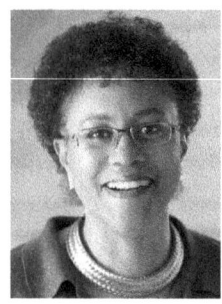

Z. Colette Edwards, MD, MBA, has been active in most segments of the healthcare arena, including, first and foremost, as a practicing gastroenterologist. She has leveraged additional training in health and wellness coaching at the Maryland University of Integrative Health and in health equity as a member of the NIH Scholars Program in translational health disparities.

Over the course of her career, she has served in a variety of roles in her quest to make a difference in the lives, health, and well-being outcomes of patients. They include being the associate medical director of a multispecialty group practice and serving in health plan medical roles. Her work has also encompassed positions at two Fortune 50 companies, including as the national medical lead for health disparities, with an initiative that won a national innovation award and as a corporate medical executive for employee health and well-being, with a multiyear record of national awards won by the team: NBGH Best Employers for Healthy Lifestyles, top 10 ranking in the "Healthiest 100 Workplaces in America," Gold status in the AHA's Workplace Health Achievement Index, and a citation for Excellence in Mental Health.

Dr. Edwards is the managing editor of the *Wharton Healthcare Quarterly*, the author of *Be Less Stressed* and a McGraw-Hill GI text, and she is a member of the board of two nonprofits, Bread for the City and T1D Exchange.

About Bold Story Press

Bold Story Press is a curated, woman-owned hybrid publishing company with a mission of publishing well-written stories by women. If your book is chosen for publication, our team of expert editors and designers will work with you to publish a professionally edited and designed book. Every woman has a story to tell. If you have written yours and want to explore publishing with Bold Story Press, contact us at https://boldstorypress.com.

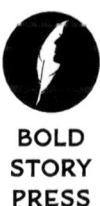

BOLD STORY PRESS

The Bold Story Press logo, designed by Grace Arsenault, was inspired by the nom de plume, or pen name, a sad necessity at one time for female authors who wanted to publish. The woman's face hidden in the quill is the profile of Virginia Woolf, who, in addition to being an early feminist writer, founded and ran her own publishing company, Hogarth Press.

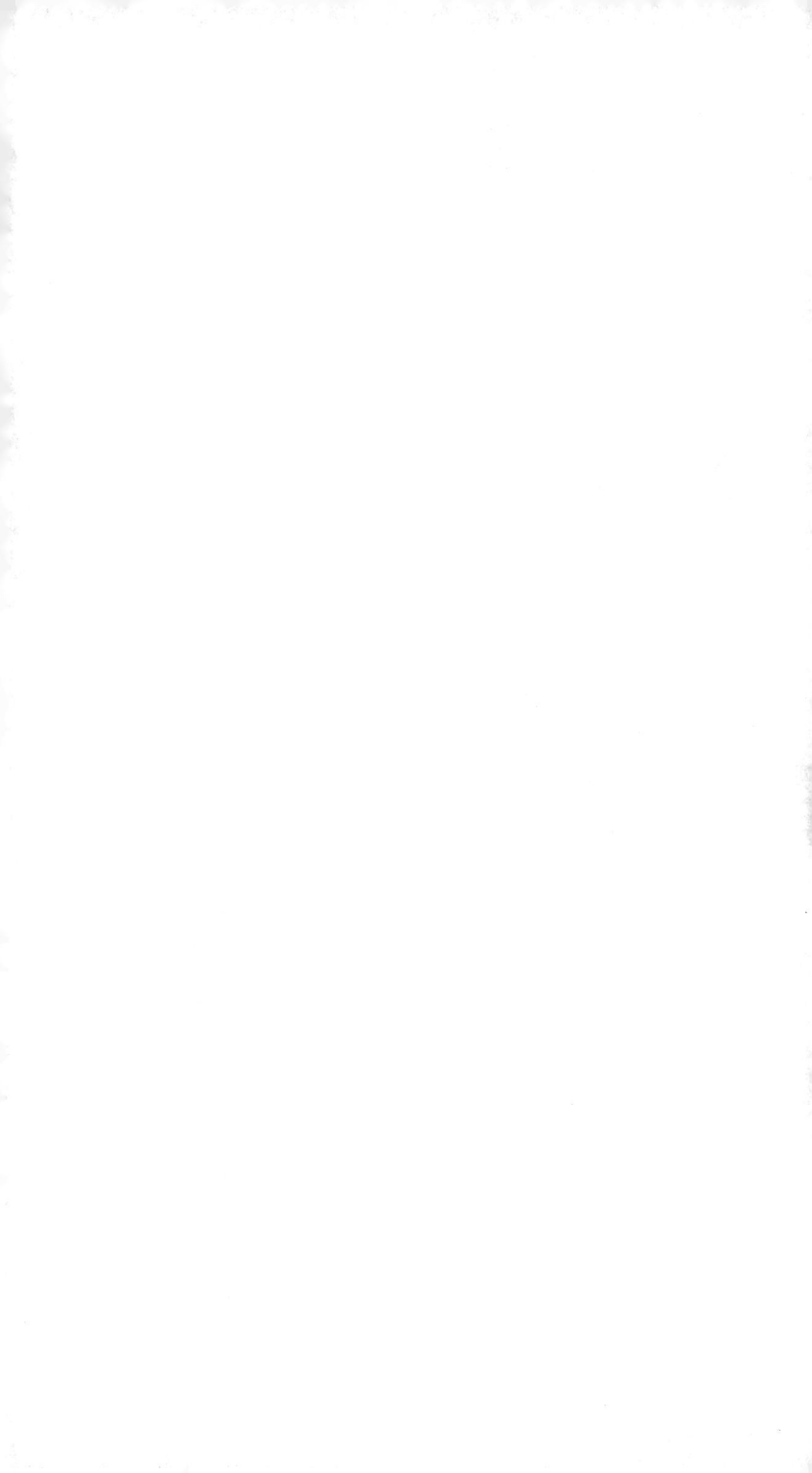

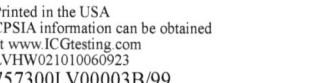
Printed in the USA
CPSIA information can be obtained
at www.ICGtesting.com
LVHW021010060923
757300LV00003B/99